I0843479

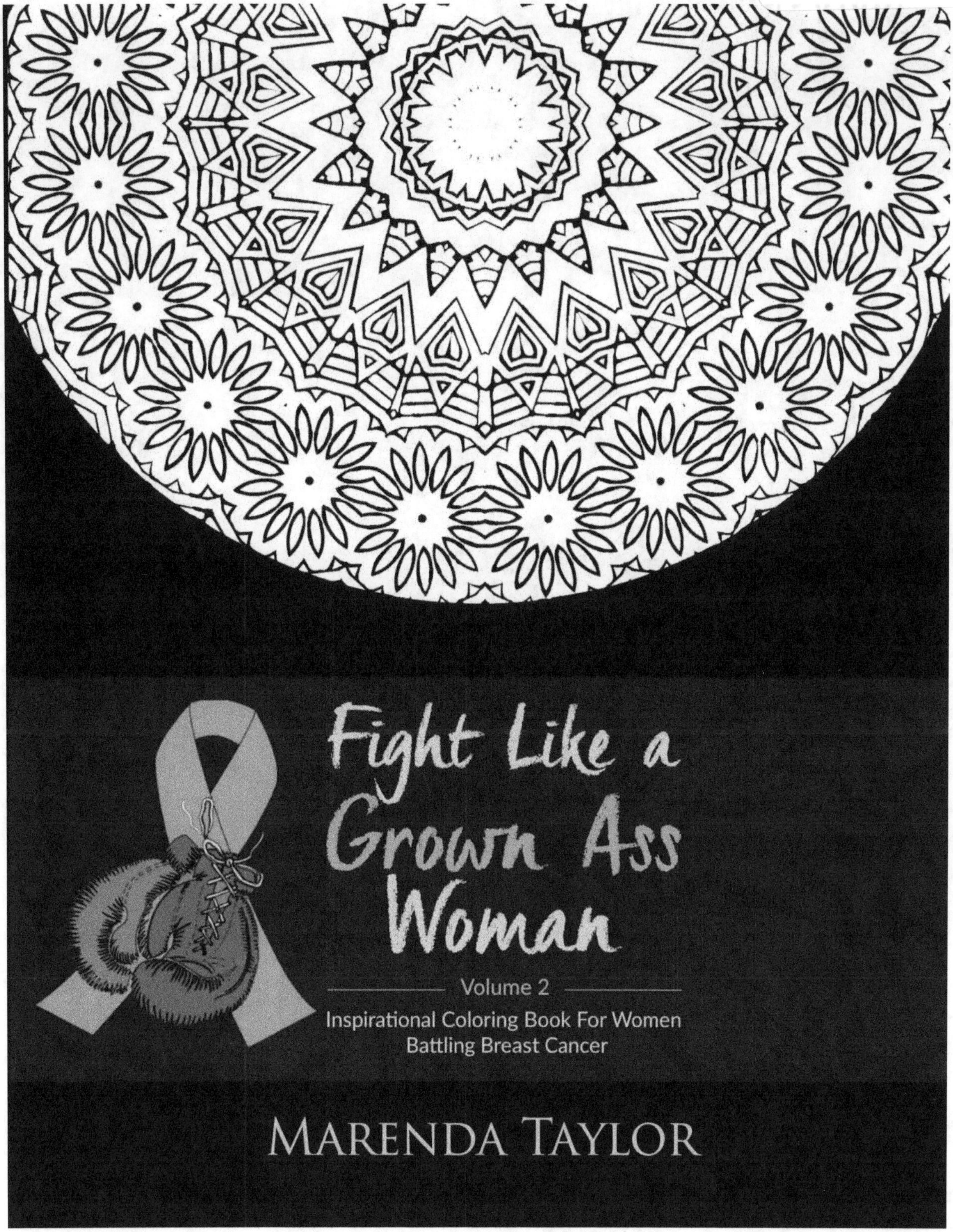

Fight Like a Grown Ass Woman

Volume 2

Inspirational Coloring Book For Women
Battling Breast Cancer

MARENDA TAYLOR

FightLikeaGrownAssWoman.com

FightLikeaGrownAssWoman.com

© 2019 MarendaTaylor.com

All rights reserved. No part of this publication may be reproduced, stored in a retrieval system, or transmitted in any form or by any means - electronic, mechanical, photocopy, recording, scanning, or other - except for brief quotations, without the prior written permission of the author.

MarendaTaylor.com has tried to trace ownership of the quotes in this book through Internet research. We regret any errors and will make any verified corrections brought to our attention in future editions.
ISBN- 9781793430311

Printed in the United States of America

FightLikeaGrownAssWoman.com

FightLikeaGrownAssWoman.com

PURPOSE

The stress of a cancer diagnosis can be extremely overwhelming. This distinguished coloring book created by a breast cancer **survivor** for breast cancer survivors, uses basic to intricate meditative designs with inspirational messages and grayscale photos of actual survivors to encourage you as well as help you **cope** with all that comes with your breast cancer journey. You are never alone! You have **Survivor Sisters** around the world that have been where you are, understand what you are going through and that want you to **Fight Like a Grown Ass Woman!** Coloring in this relaxing adult coloring book is one of many ways to fight! As you begin coloring the pages in this book it will help you tame monkey mind, reduce stress, lower anxiety, decrease negative emotions, and maintain a positive attitude while fueling your **fighting spirit** inspiring you to **live** every day of your life abundantly.

FightLikeaGrownAssWoman.com

SUPPORT the fighters

ADMIRE the survivors

REMEMBER the angels

FightLikeaGrownAssWoman.com

FightLikeaGrownAssWoman.com

Dedicated to my paternal grandmother Eleanor Wise Hughes Penn, the brave courageous ladies in my breast cancer *support group* at **Cancer Support Community Redondo Beach** and <u>ALL</u> *Breast Cancer Survivors*. #SurvivorSisters

IN LOVING MEMORY OF

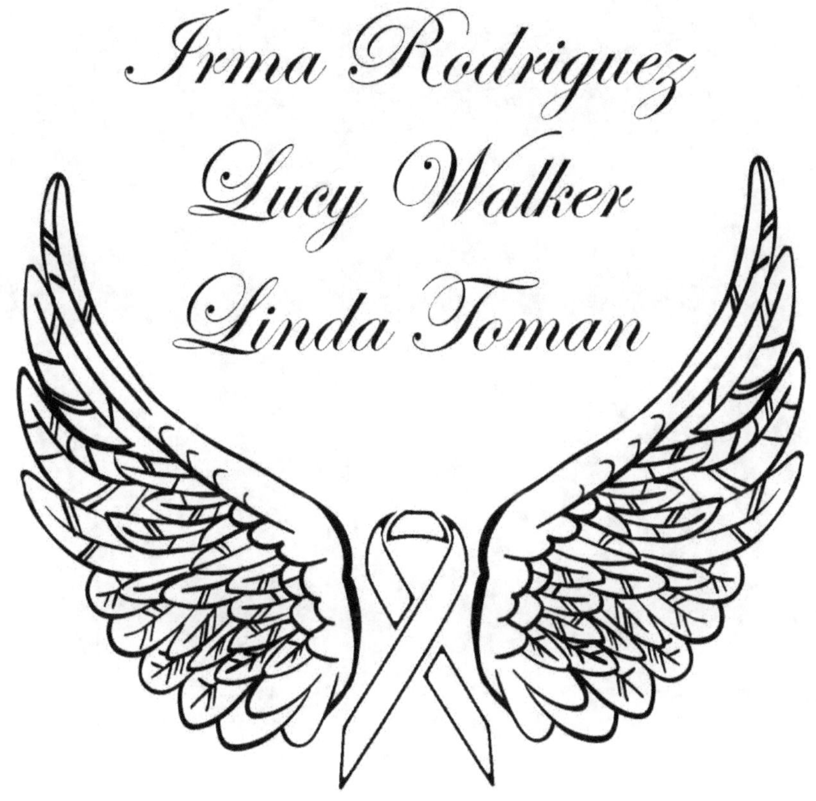

FightLikeaGrownAssWoman.com

FightLikeaGrownAssWoman.com

COLORING TIPS

This coloring book was strategically designed for mindfulness meditation, RELAXation, and inspiration with detailed and in some cases very elaborate designs including pages with grayscale photography.

It is suggested that you use sharpened colored pencils for the designs in this book. You may also use crayons, markers, and/or gel pens. Markers may bleed through the page.

This is your coloring book and you make the rules. You are a Grown Ass Woman… You can color in the lines, outside the lines, or draw your own lines…. **Just relax and *enjoy what I call Coloring Therapy*!**

*Follow on Instagram @FightLikeaGrownAssWoman and @MarendaTaylor share your coloring pages using the hashtags: #SurvivorSisters #ColoringTherapy #FightLikeaGrownAssWoman

FightLikeaGrownAssWoman.com

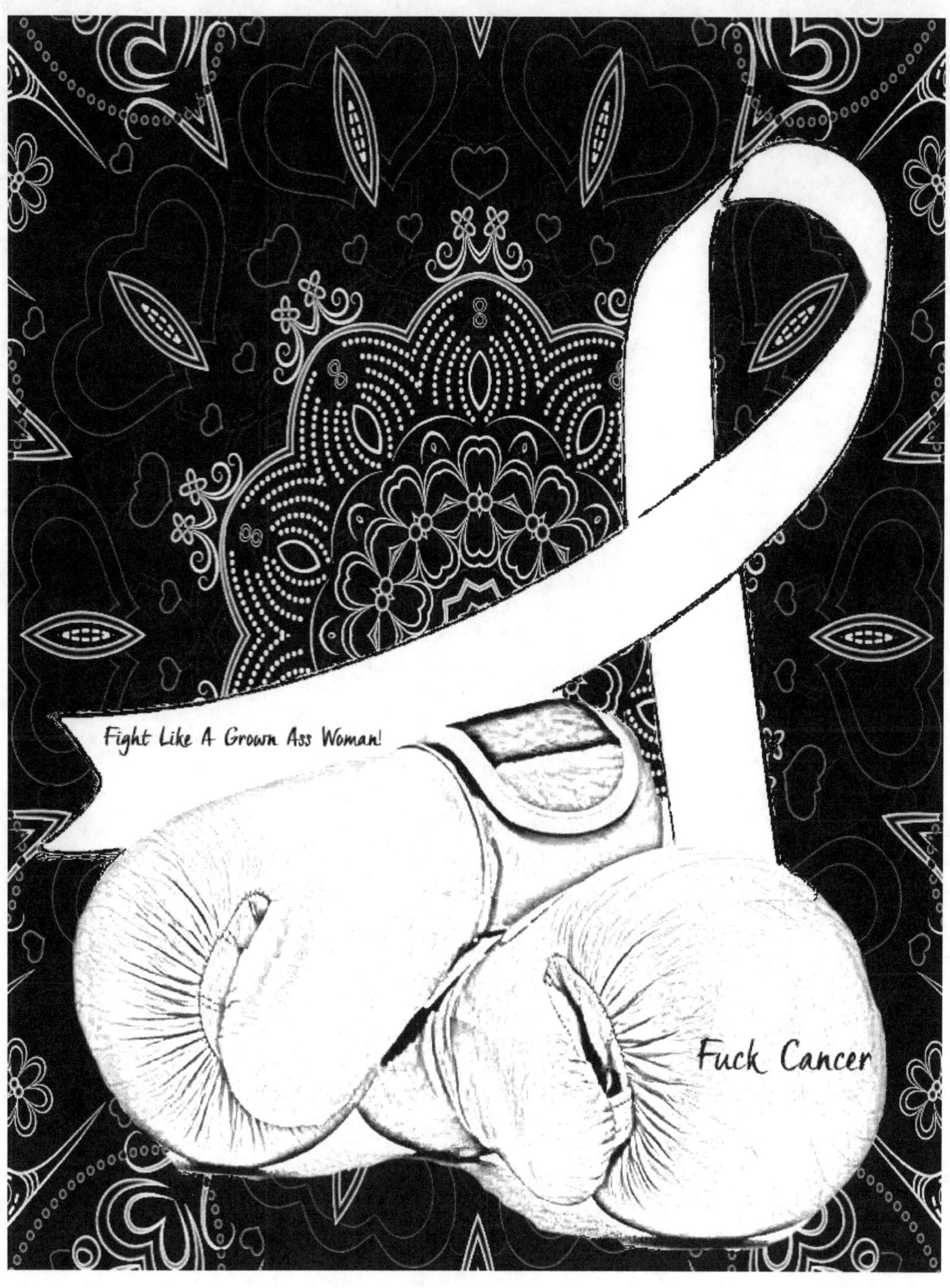

Fight Like A Grown Ass Woman!
Fuck Cancer

FightLikeaGrownAssWoman.com

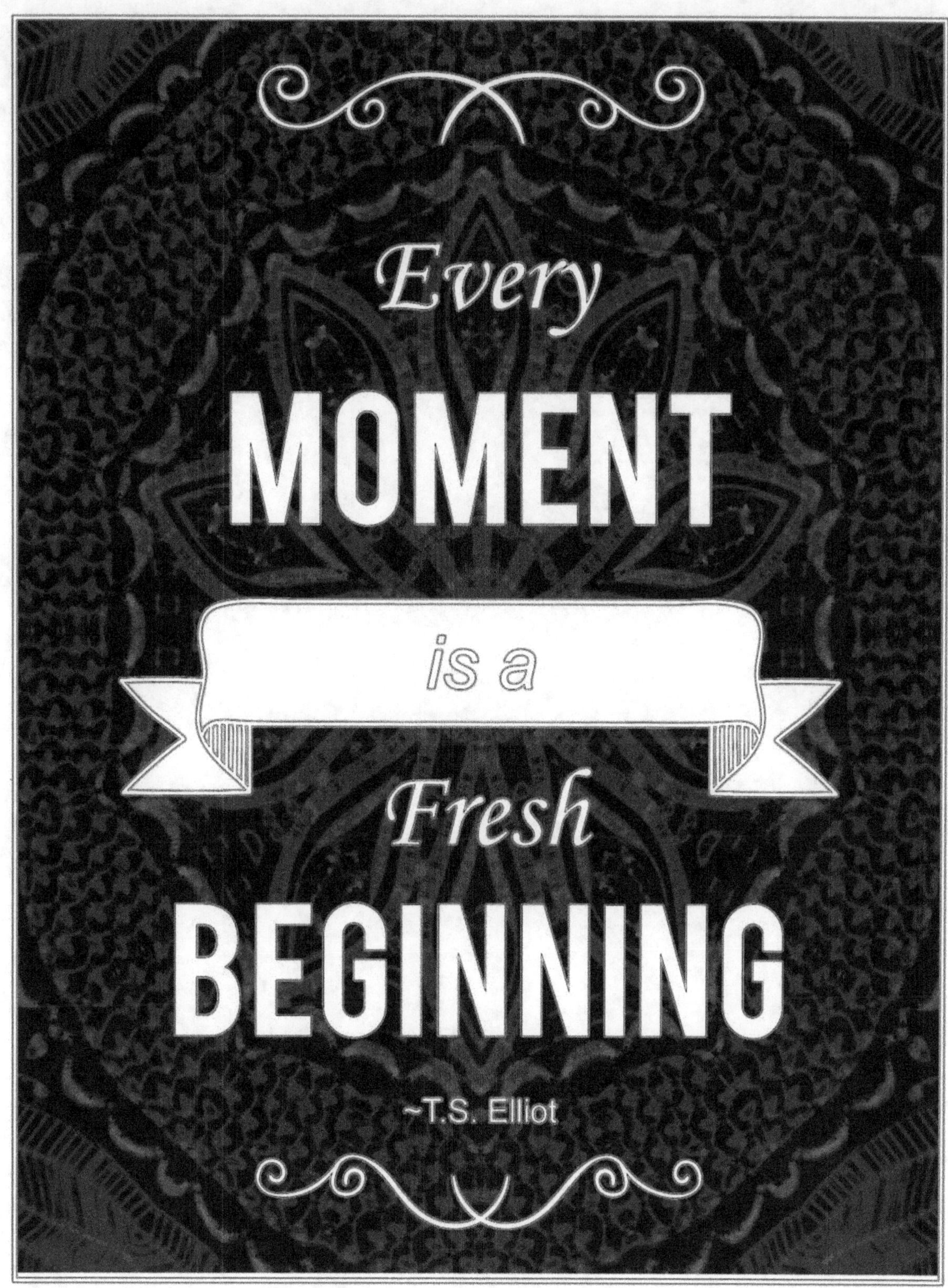

FightLikeaGrownAssWoman.com

FightLikeaGrownAssWoman.com

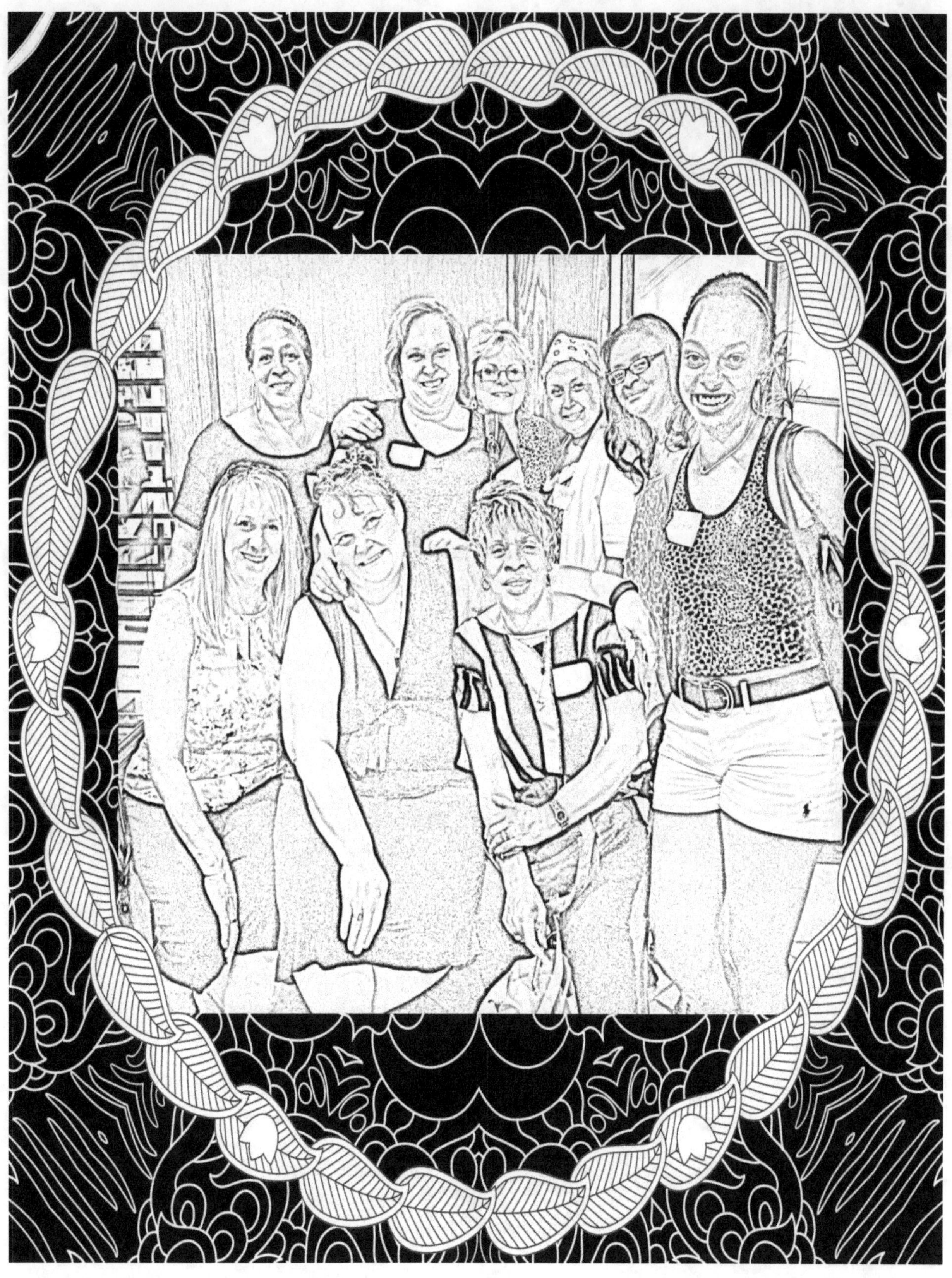

FightLikeaGrownAssWoman.com

FightLikeaGrownAssWoman.com

FightLikeaGrownAssWoman.com

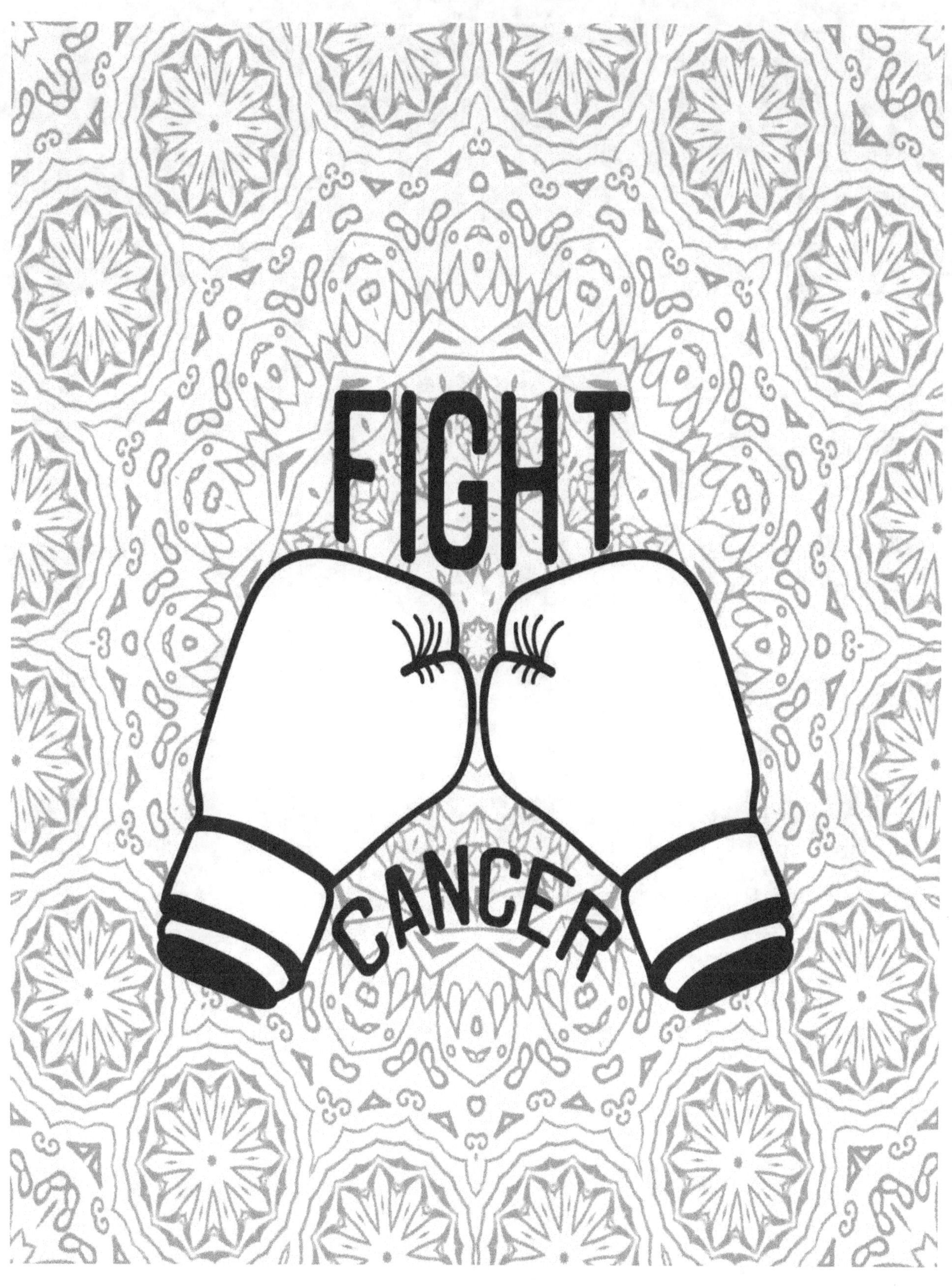

FightLikeaGrownAssWoman.com

FightLikeaGrownAssWoman.com

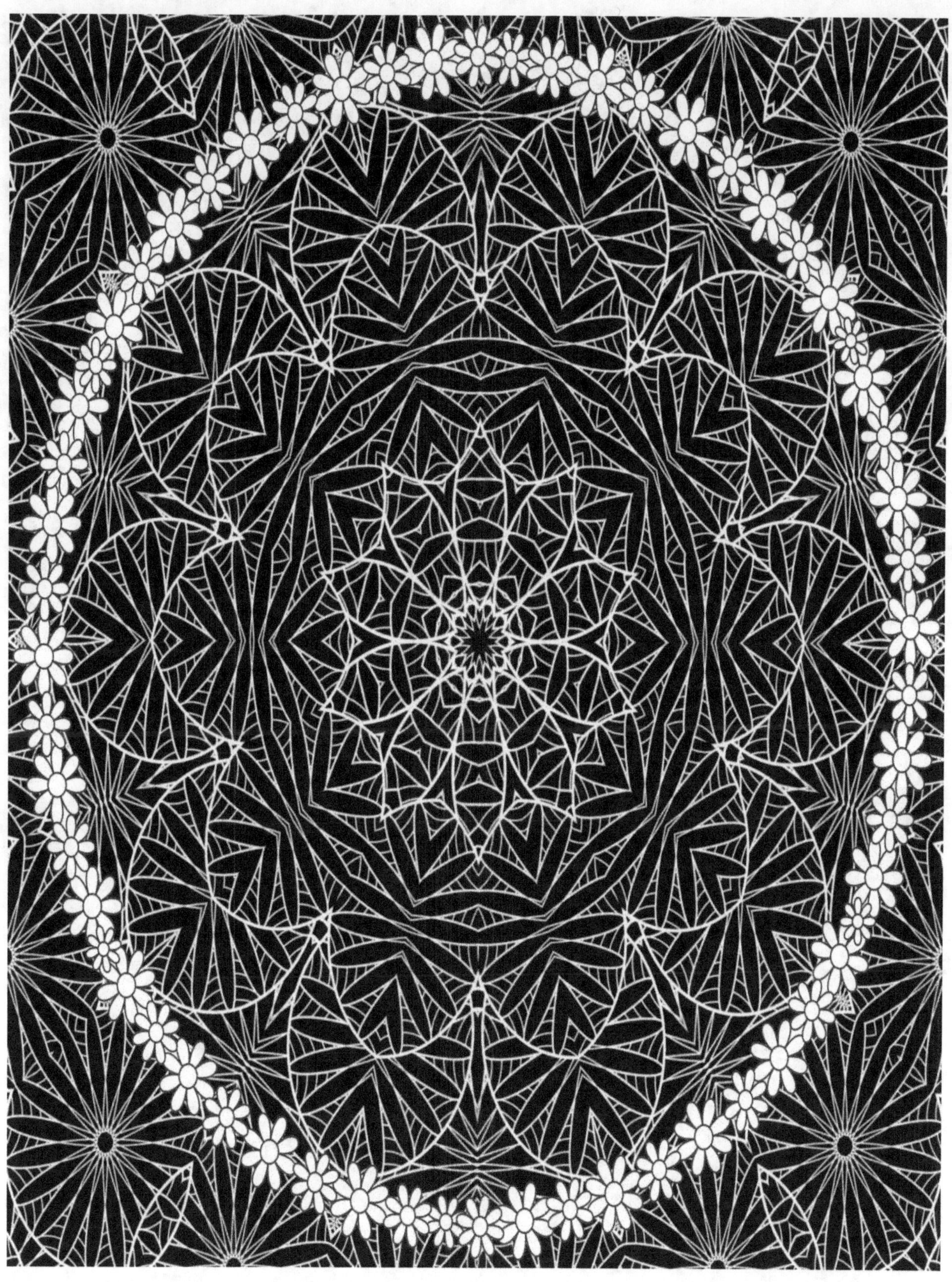

FightLikeaGrownAssWoman.com

FightLikeaGrownAssWoman.com

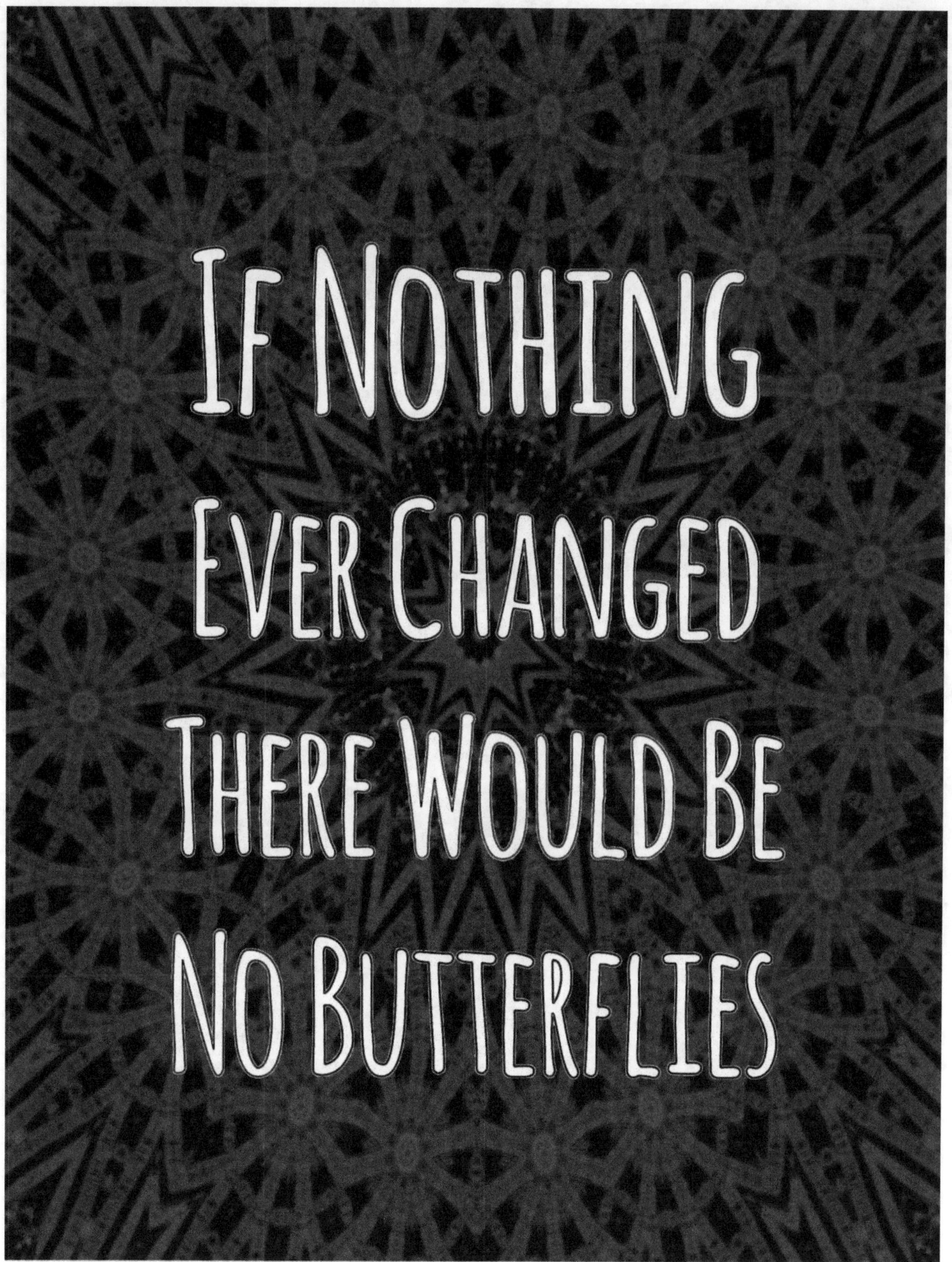

FightLikeaGrownAssWoman.com

FightLikeaGrownAssWoman.com

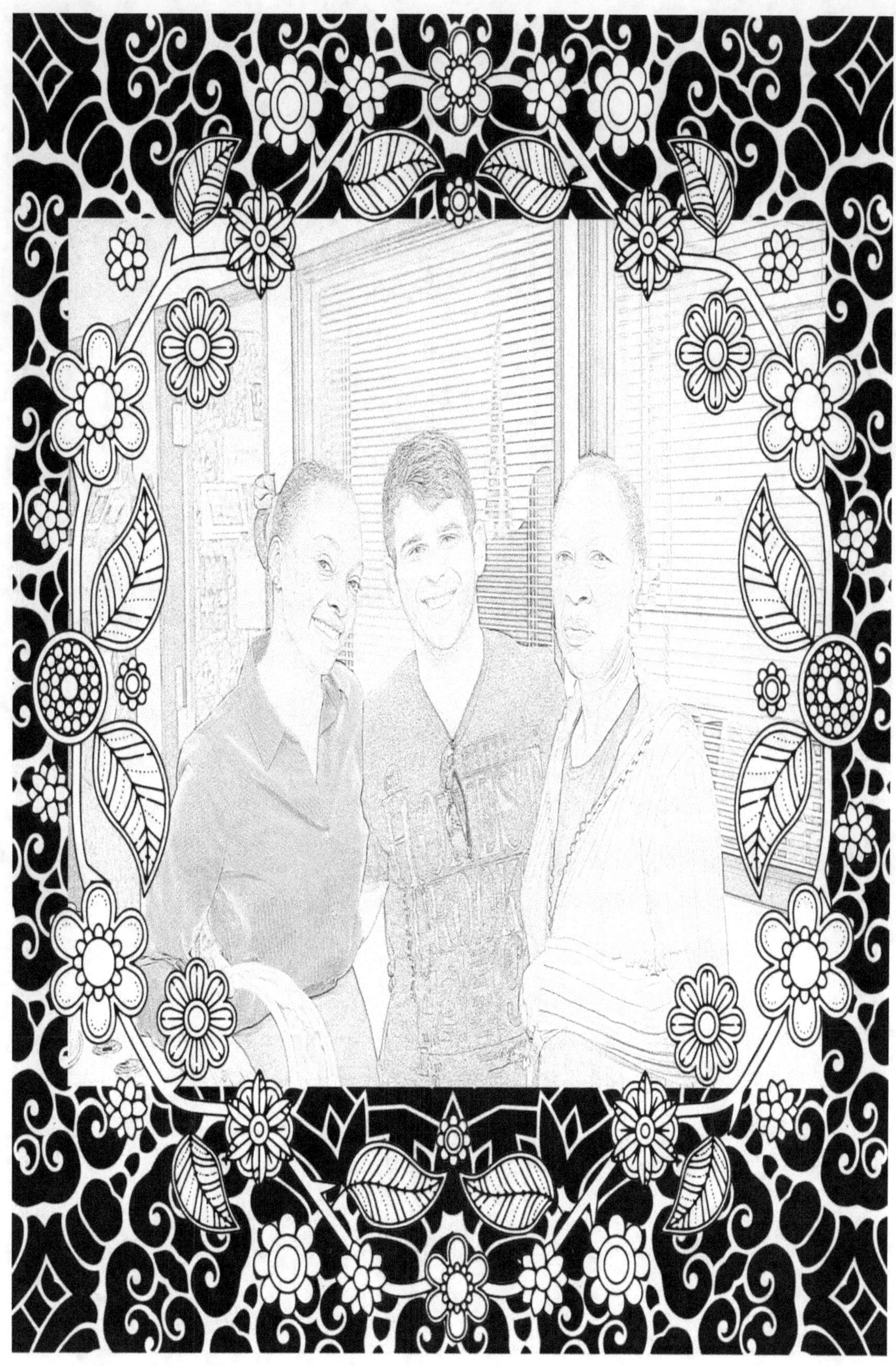

FightLikeaGrownAssWoman.com

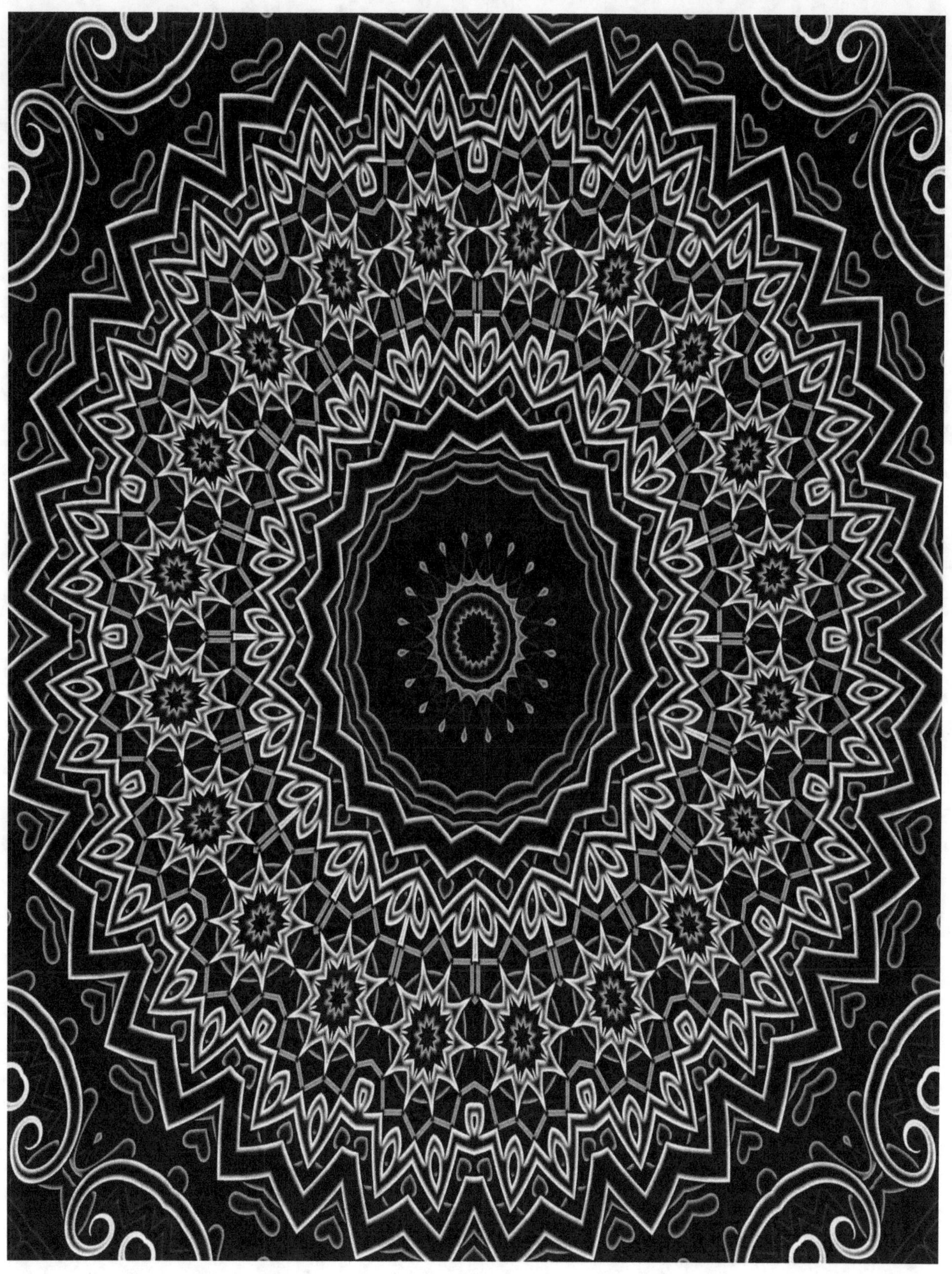

FightLikeaGrownAssWoman.com

FightLikeaGrownAssWoman.com

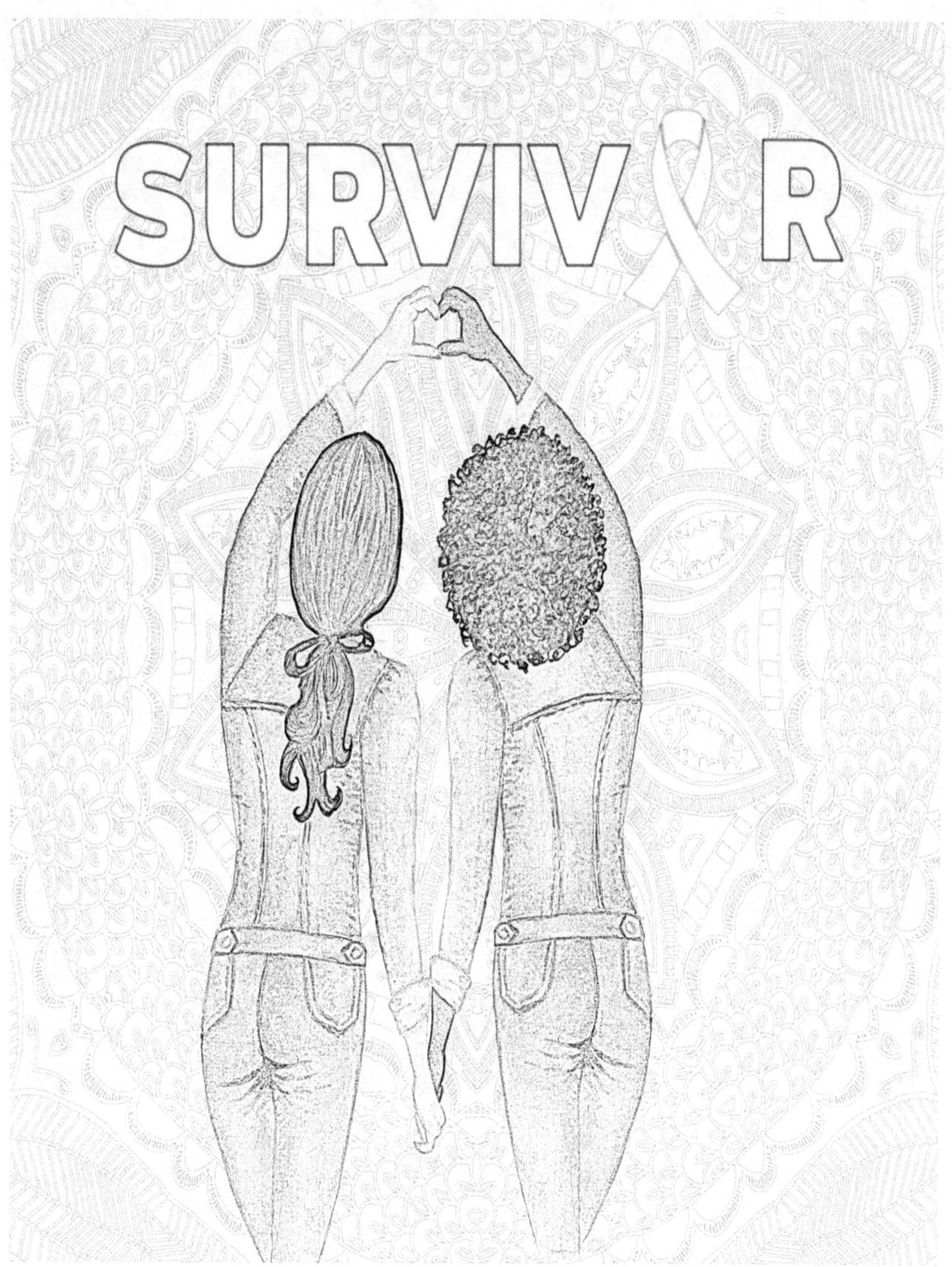

FightLikeaGrownAssWoman.com

FightLikeaGrownAssWoman.com

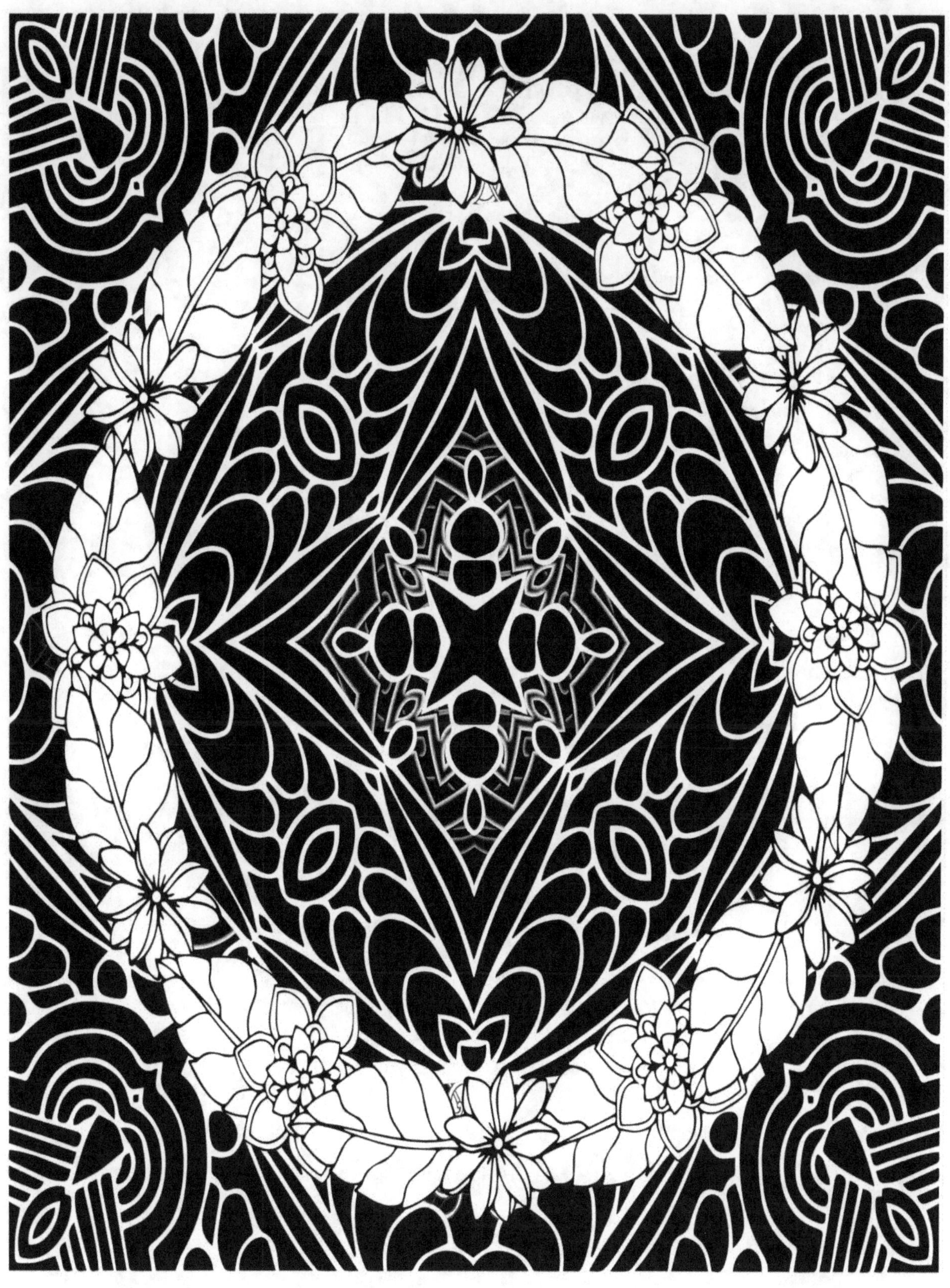

FightLikeaGrownAssWoman.com

FightLikeaGrownAssWoman.com

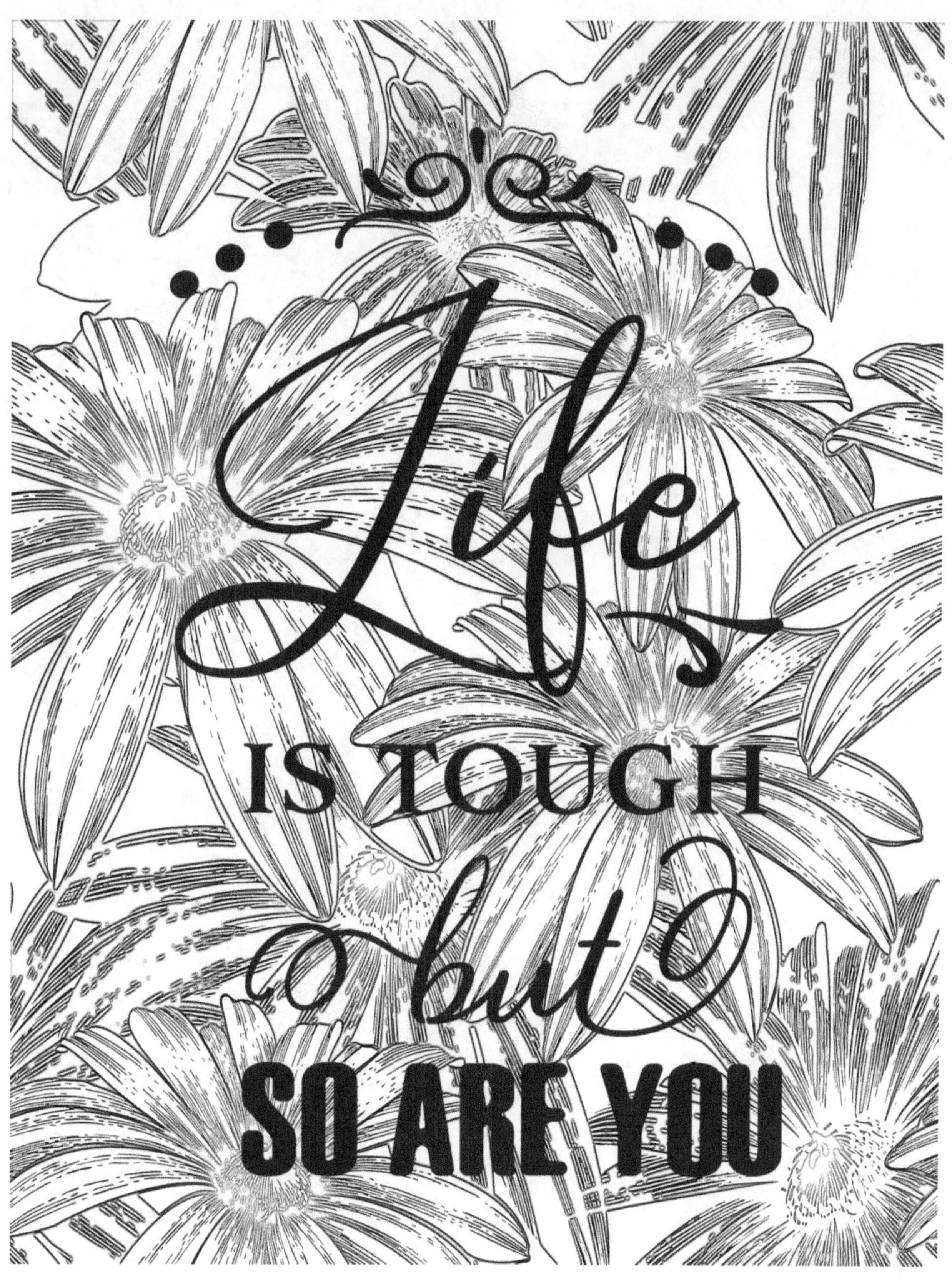

FightLikeaGrownAssWoman.com

FightLikeaGrownAssWoman.com

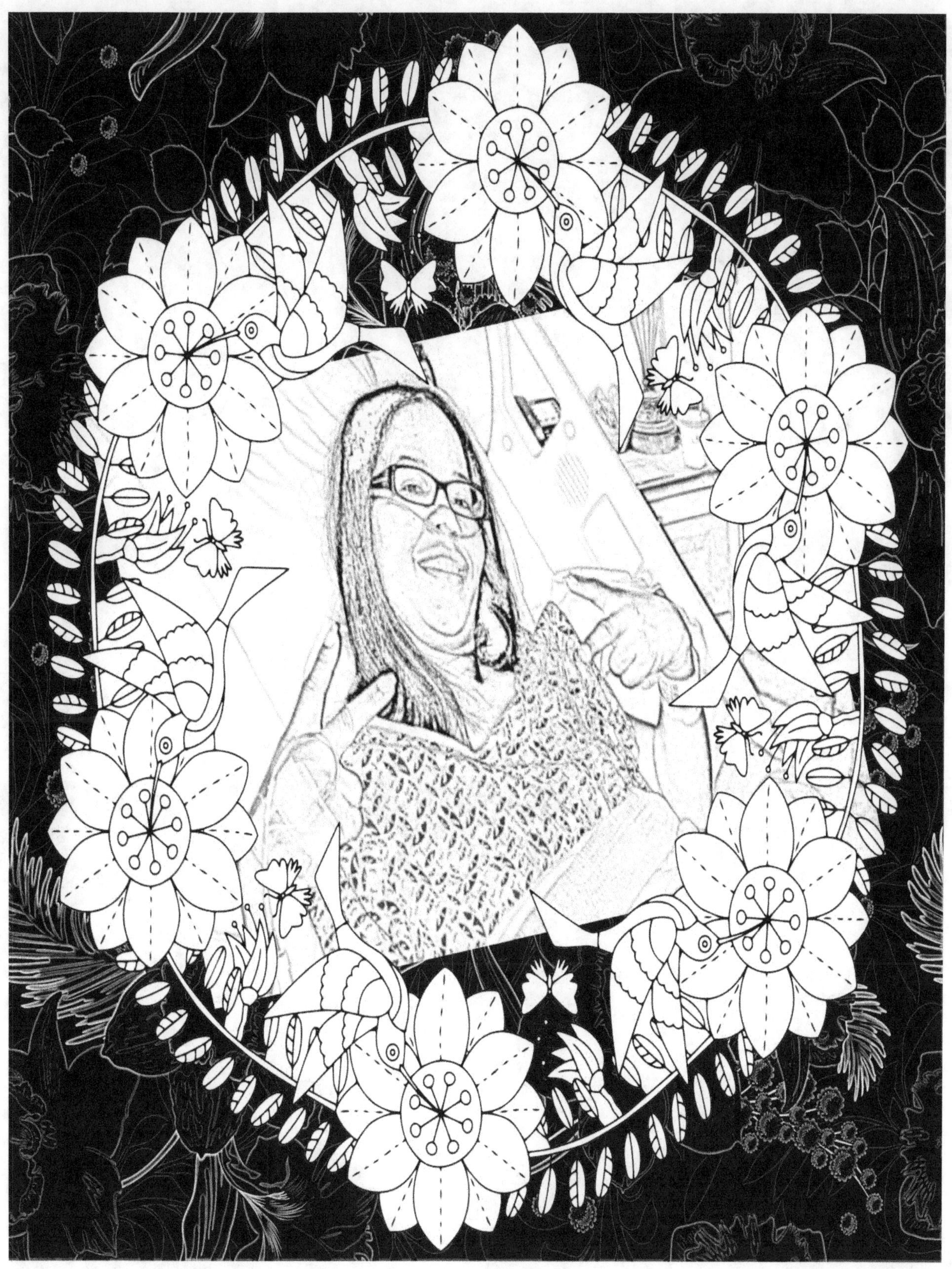

FightLikeaGrownAssWoman.com

FightLikeaGrownAssWoman.com

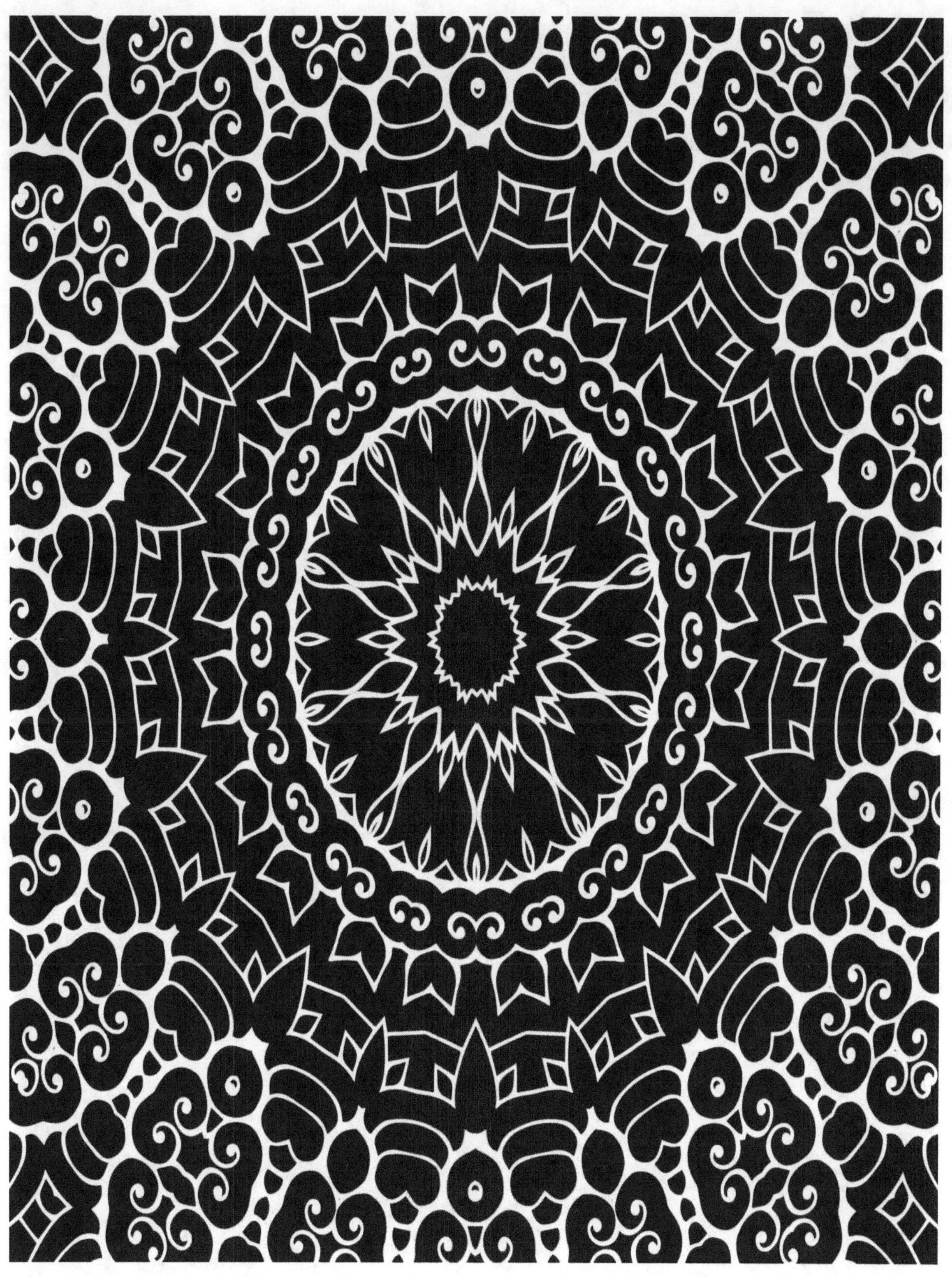

FightLikeaGrownAssWoman.com

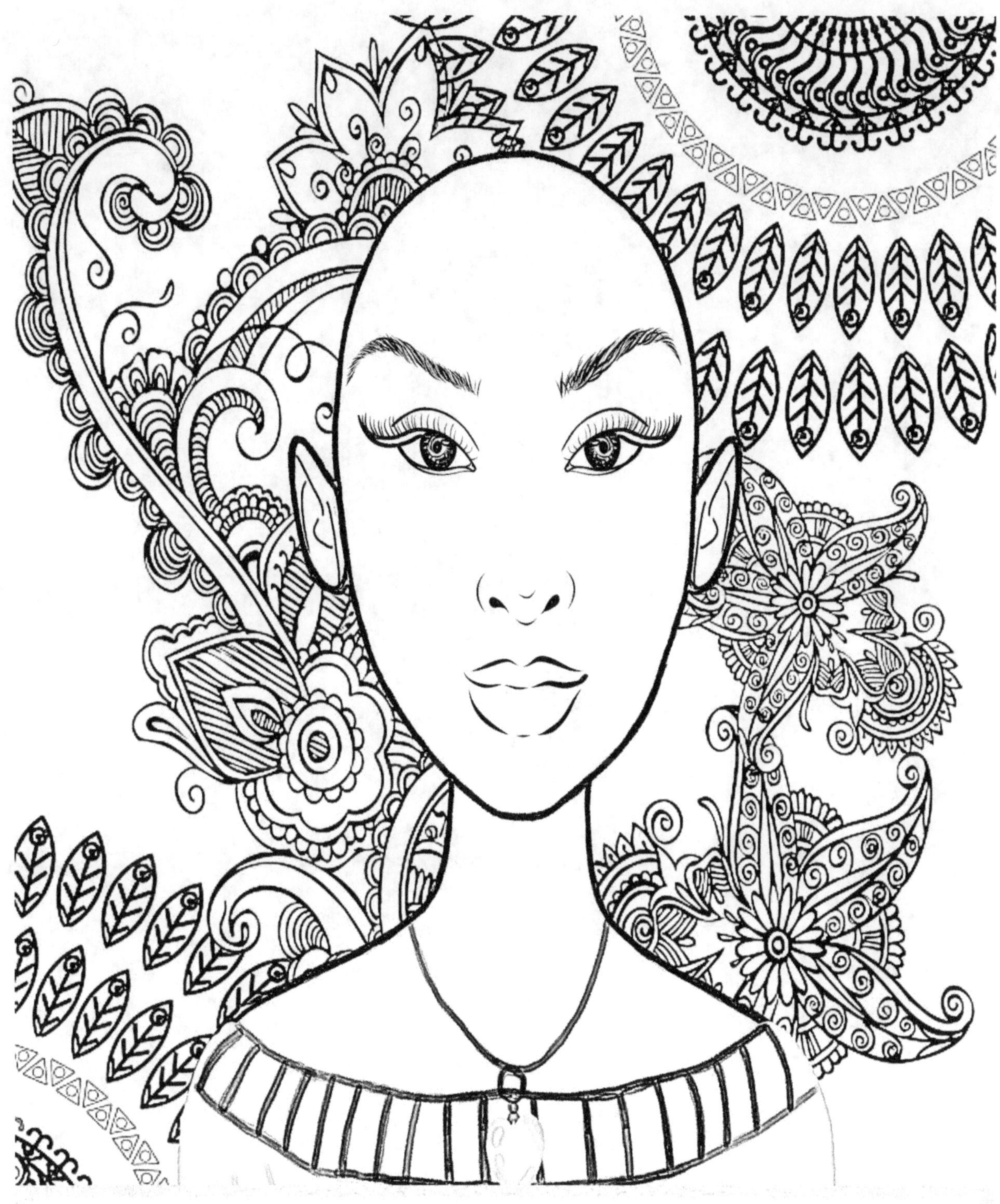

"Being challenged in life is inevitable, Being defeated is optional."
~ Roger Crawford

FightLikeaGrownAssWoman.com

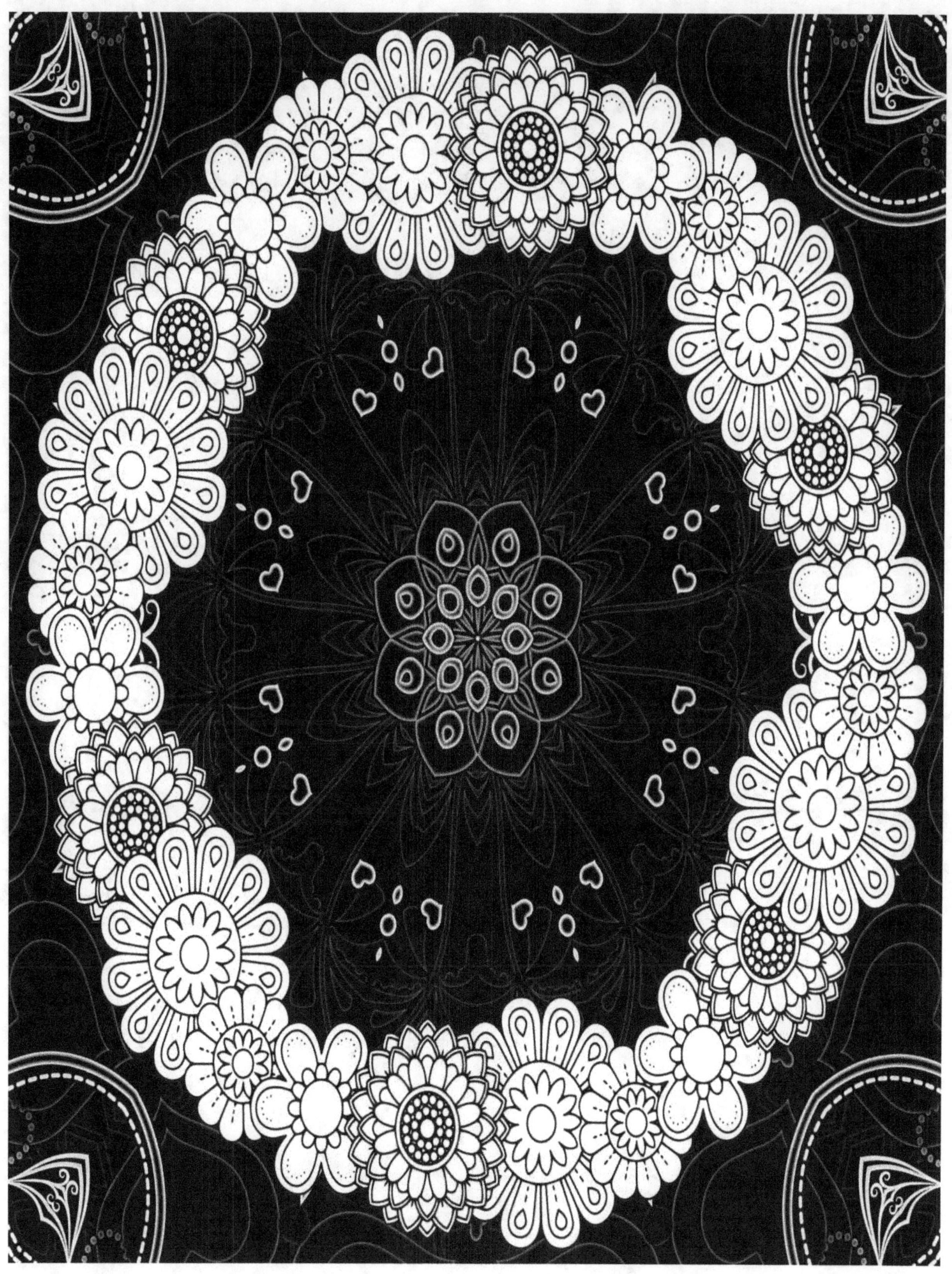

FightLikeaGrownAssWoman.com

FightLikeaGrownAssWoman.com

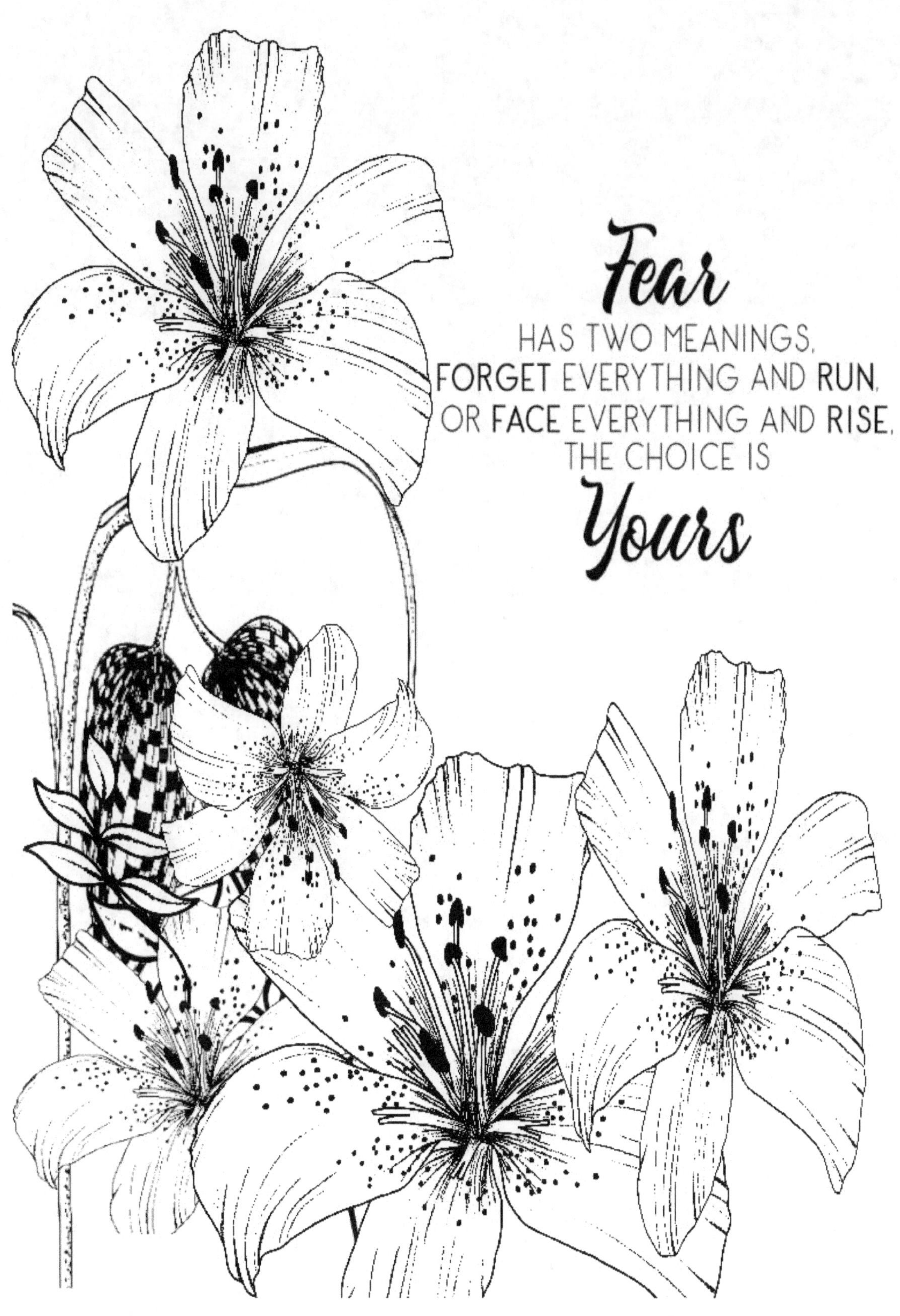

FightLikeaGrownAssWoman.com

FightLikeaGrownAssWoman.com

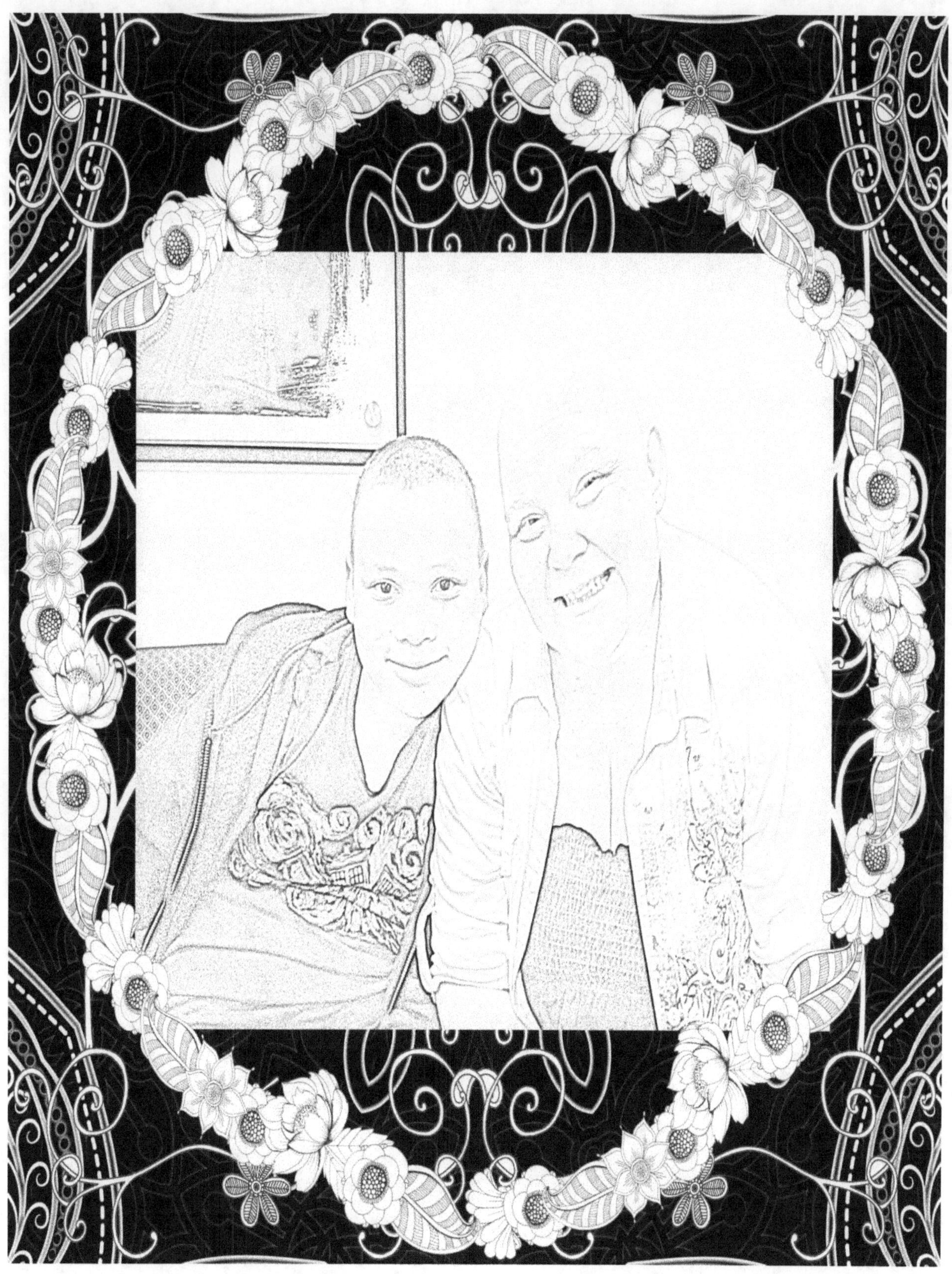

FightLikeaGrownAssWoman.com

FightLikeaGrownAssWoman.com

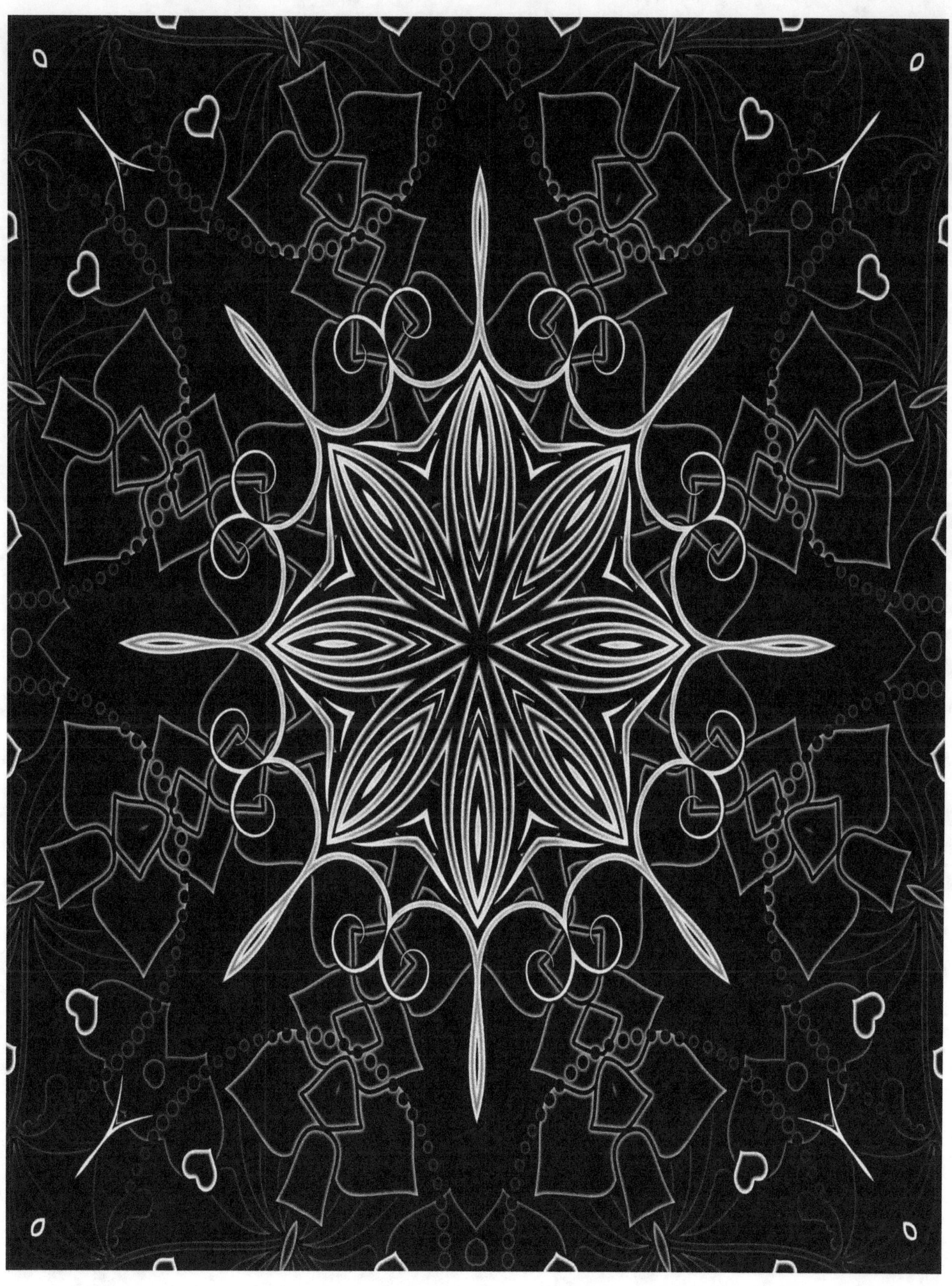

FightLikeaGrownAssWoman.com

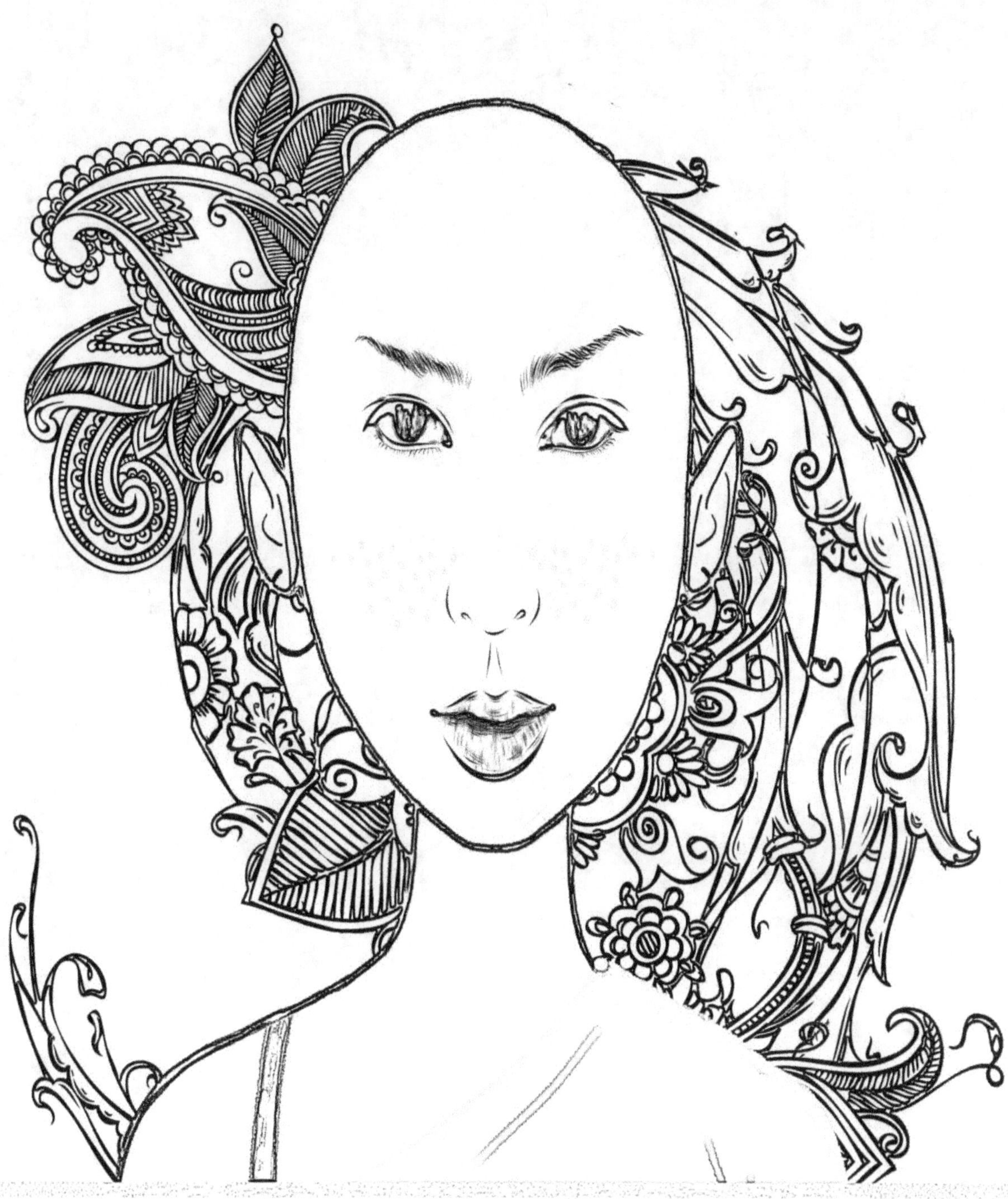

FightLikeaGrownAssWoman.com

FightLikeaGrownAssWoman.com

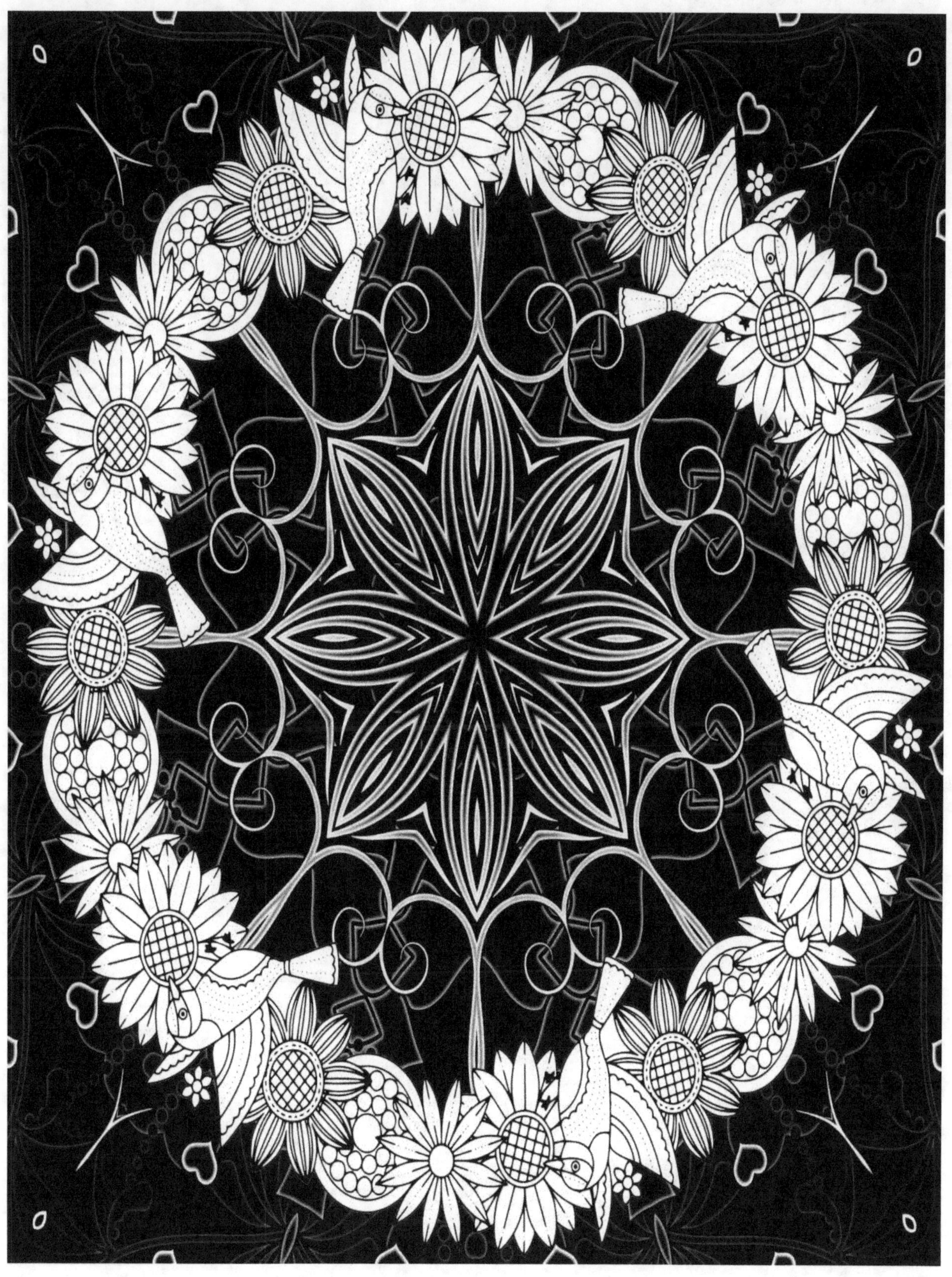

FightLikeaGrownAssWoman.com

FightLikeaGrownAssWoman.com

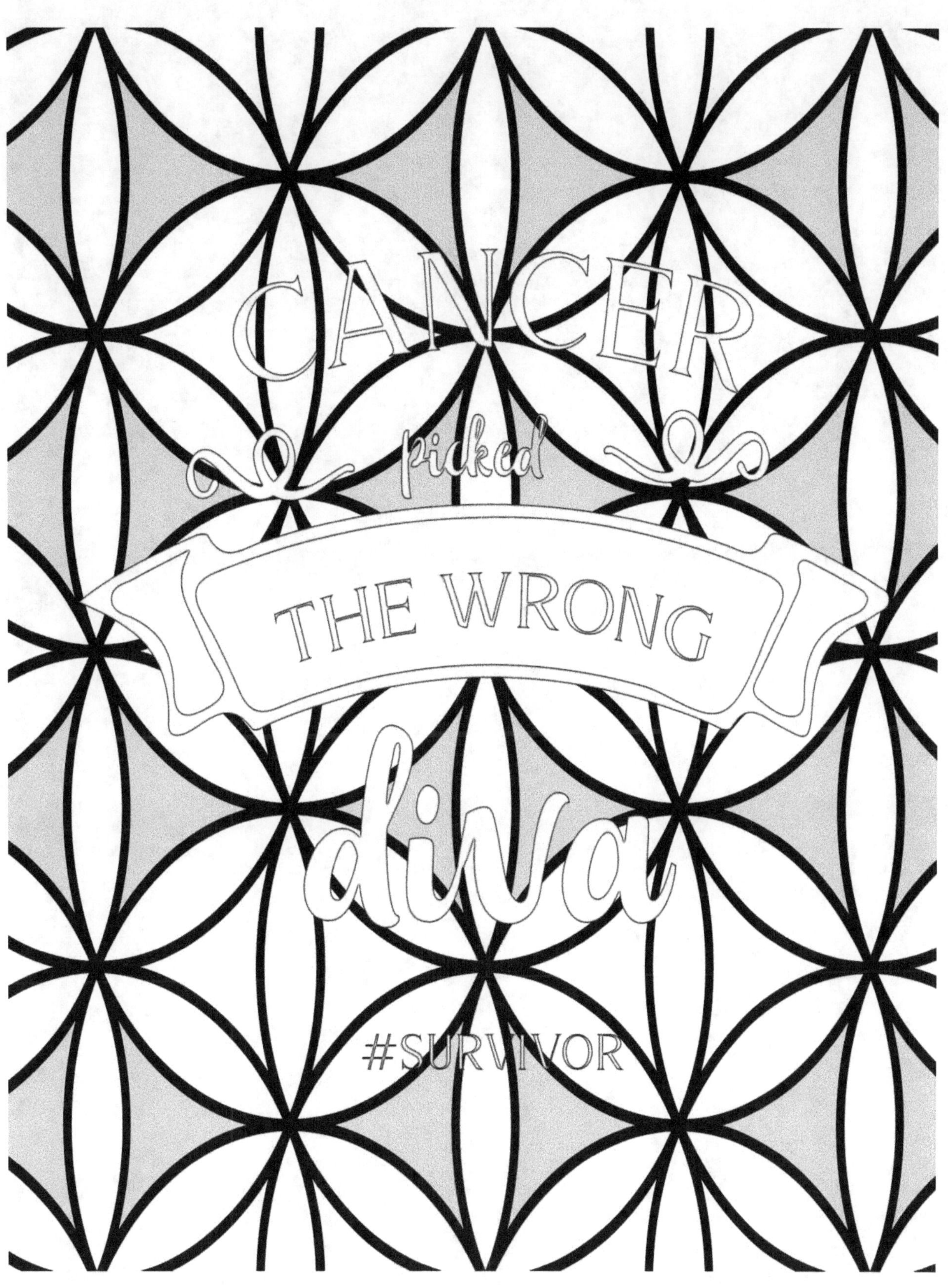

FightLikeaGrownAssWoman.com

FightLikeaGrownAssWoman.com

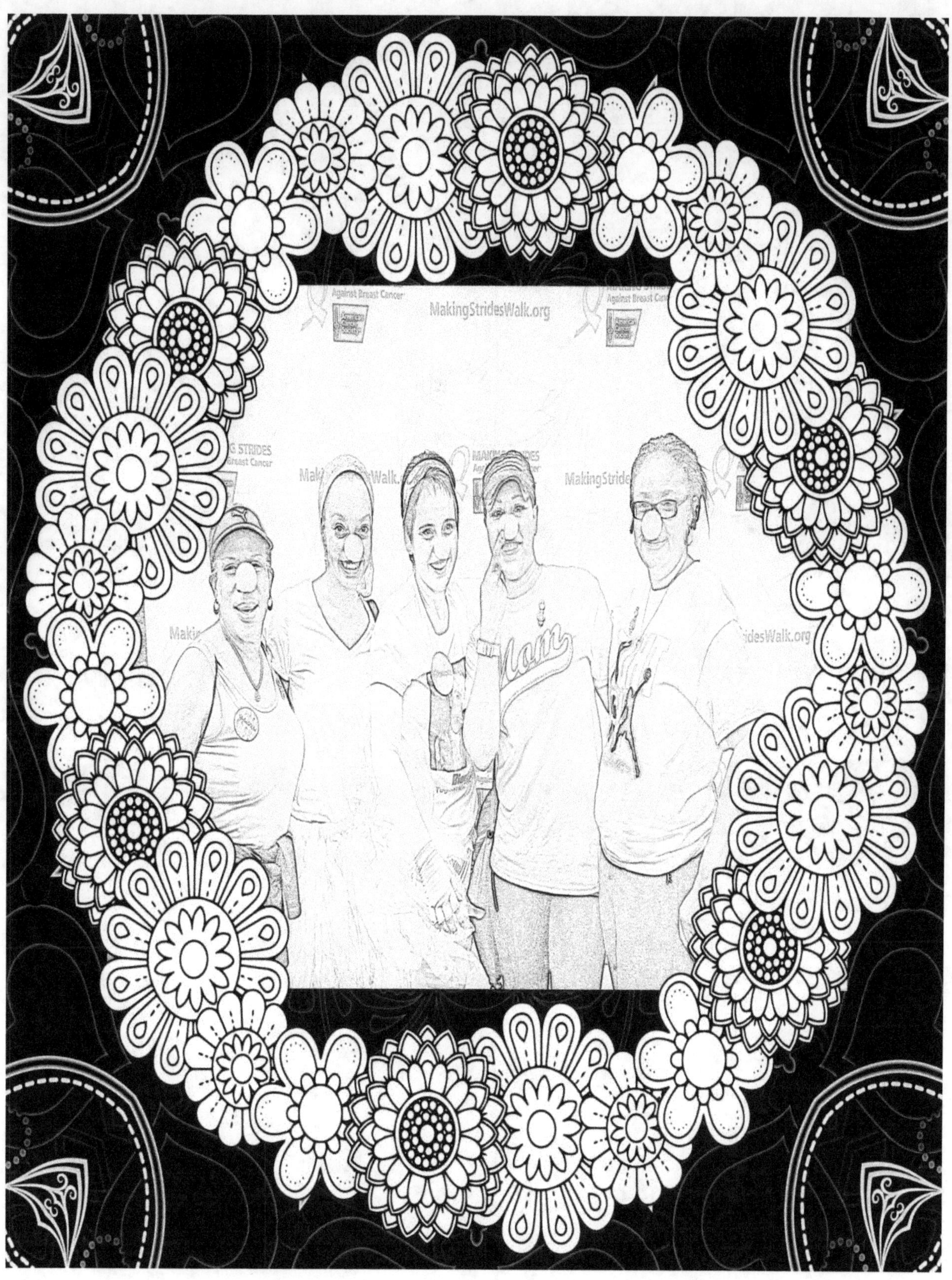

Against Breast Cancer
MakingStridesWalk.org
Against Breast Cancer
MakingStride
MakingStride
Mom

FightLikeaGrownAssWoman.com

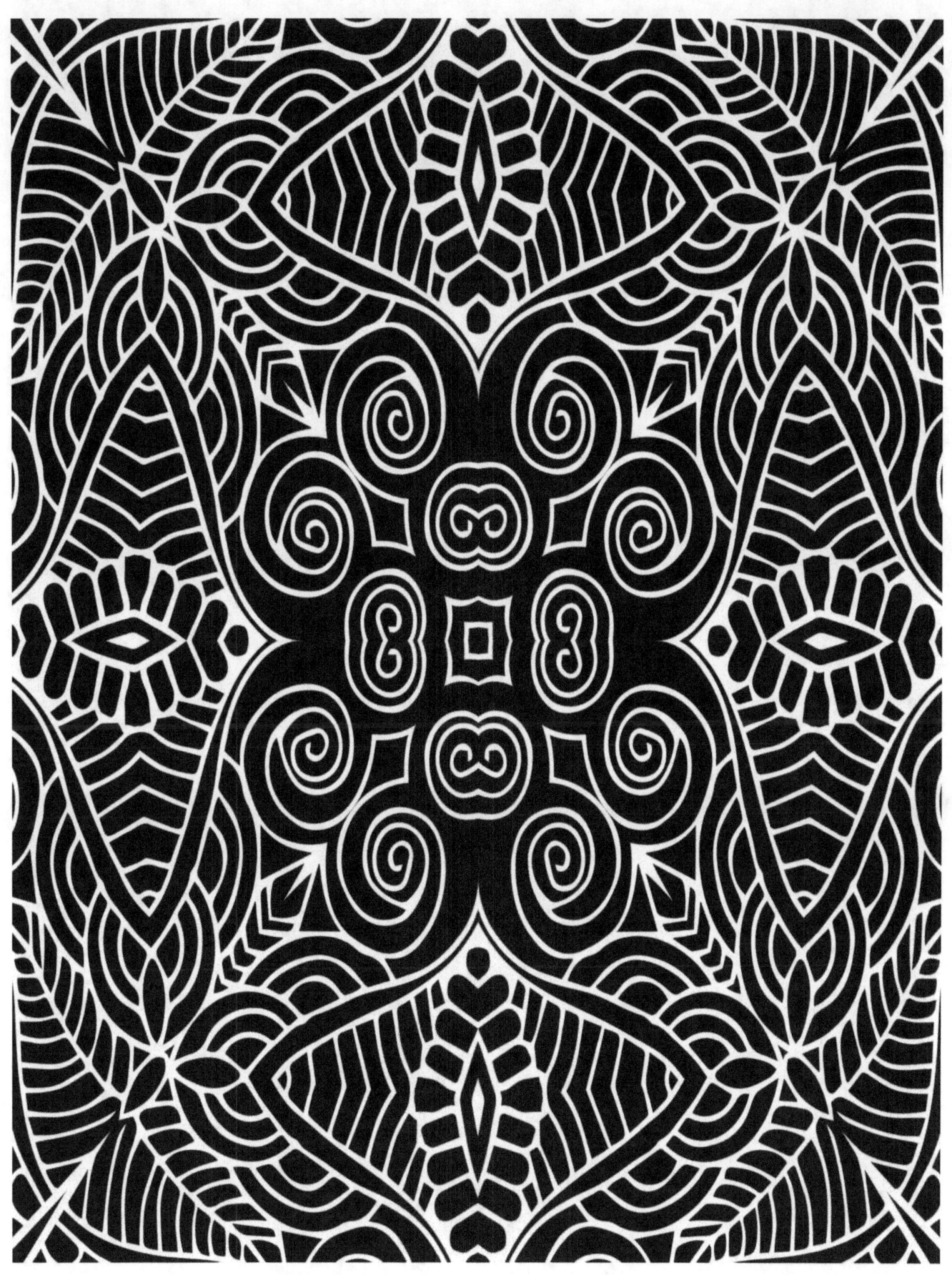

FightLikeaGrownAssWoman.com

FightLikeaGrownAssWoman.com

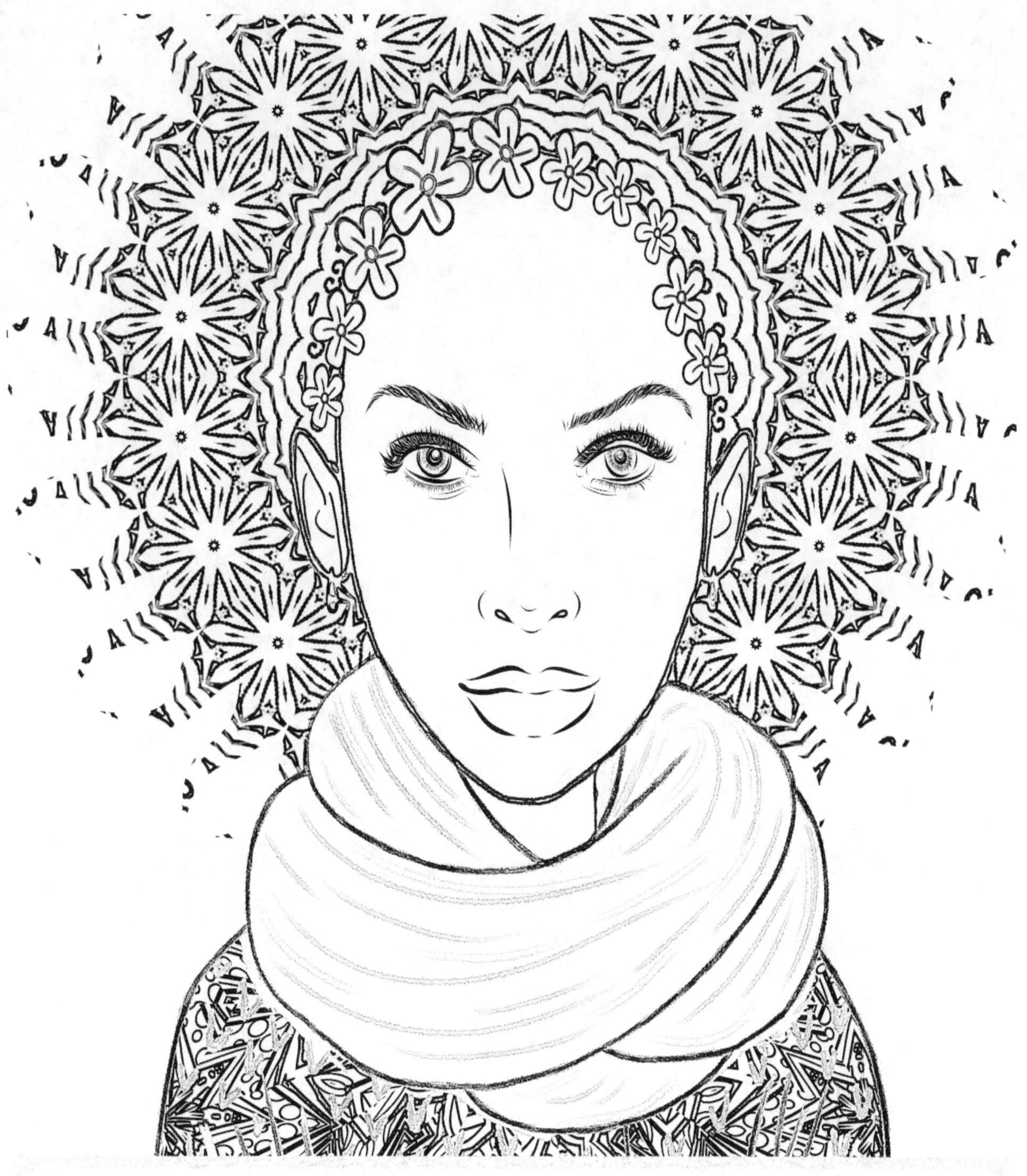

"Nothing is so strong as gentleness, nothing so gentle as real strength."
~ Saint Francis de Sales

FightLikeaGrownAssWoman.com

FightLikeaGrownAssWoman.com

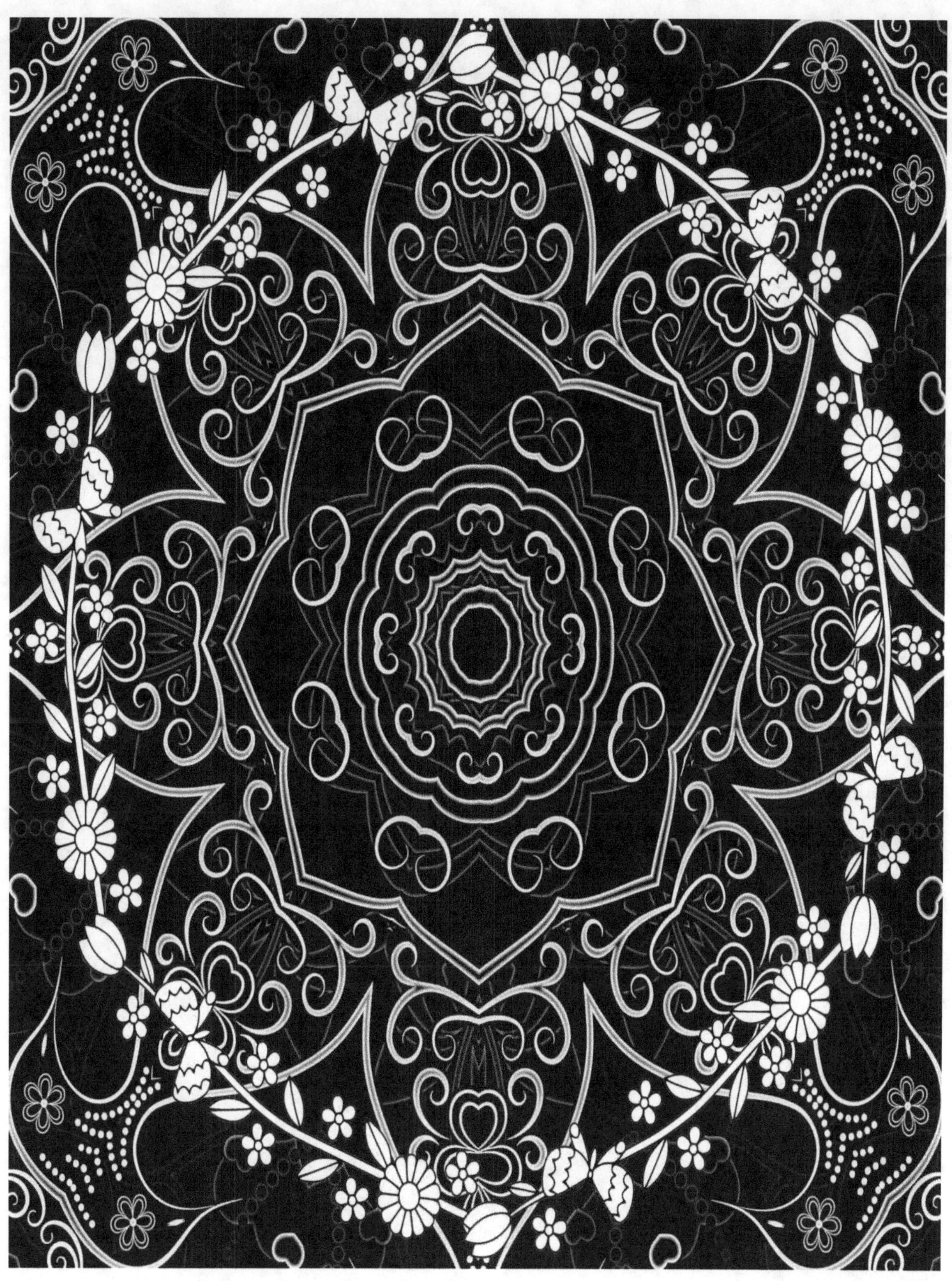

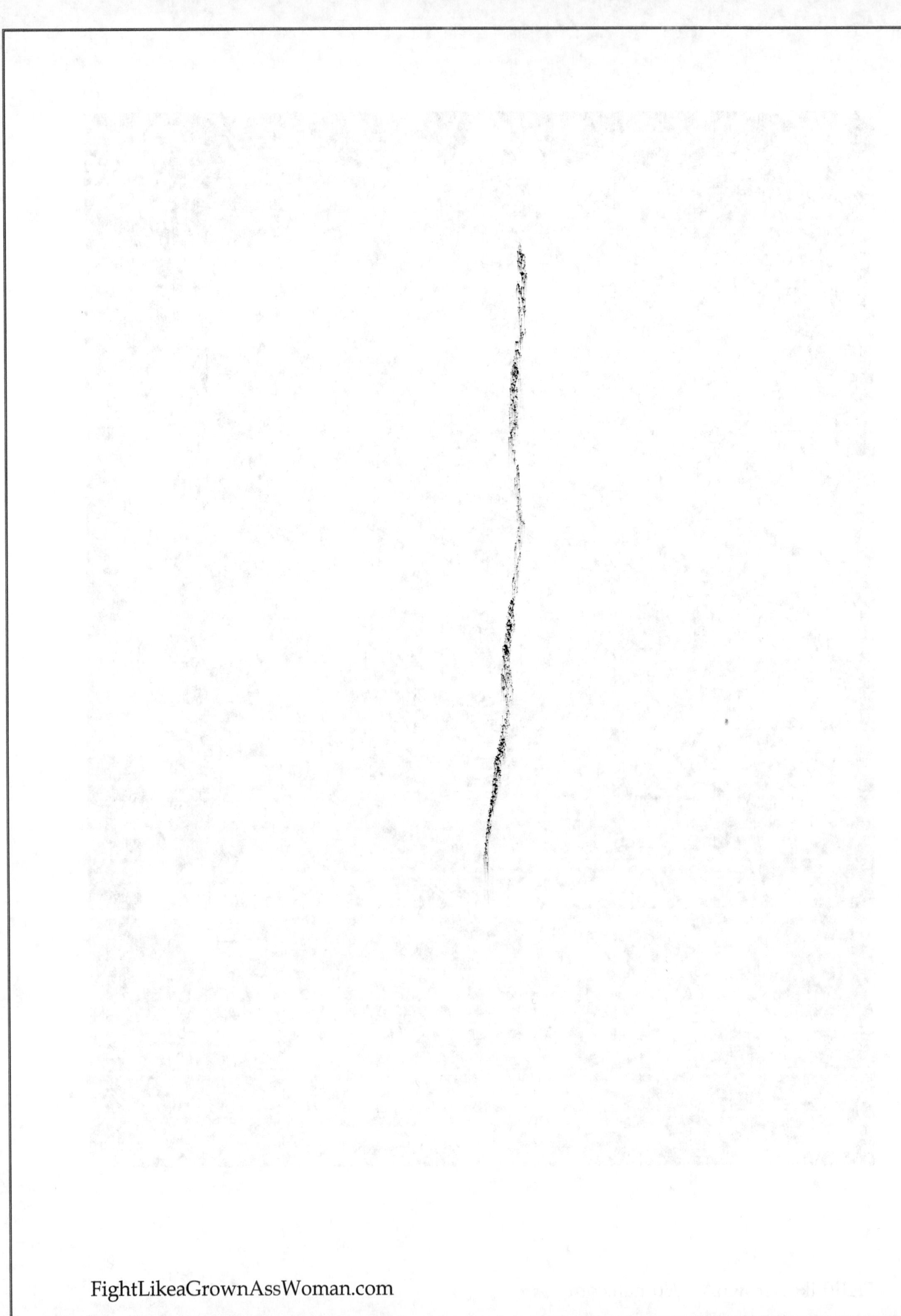

FightLikeaGrownAssWoman.com

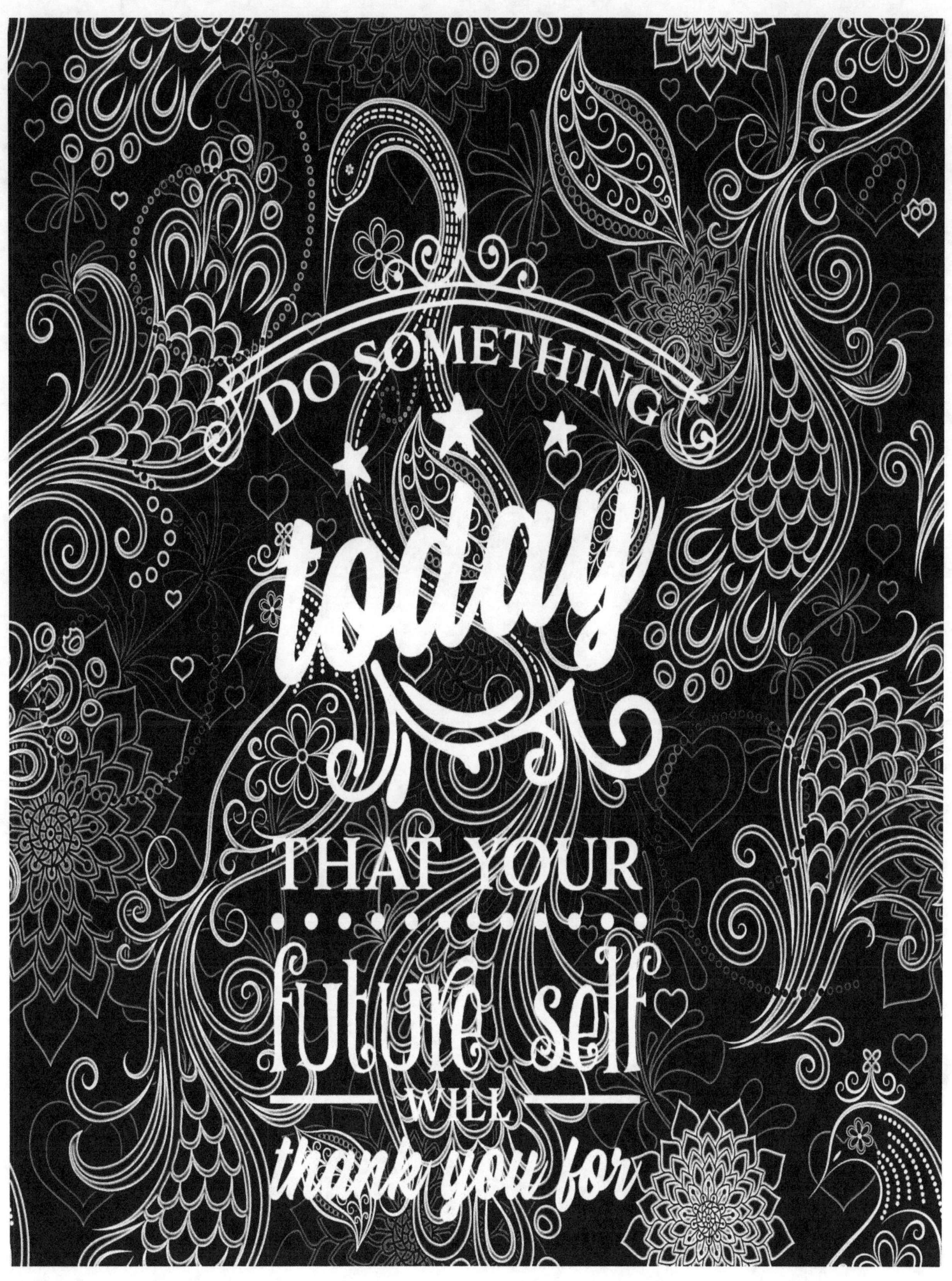

DO SOMETHING
today
THAT YOUR
future self
WILL
thank you for

FightLikeaGrownAssWoman.com

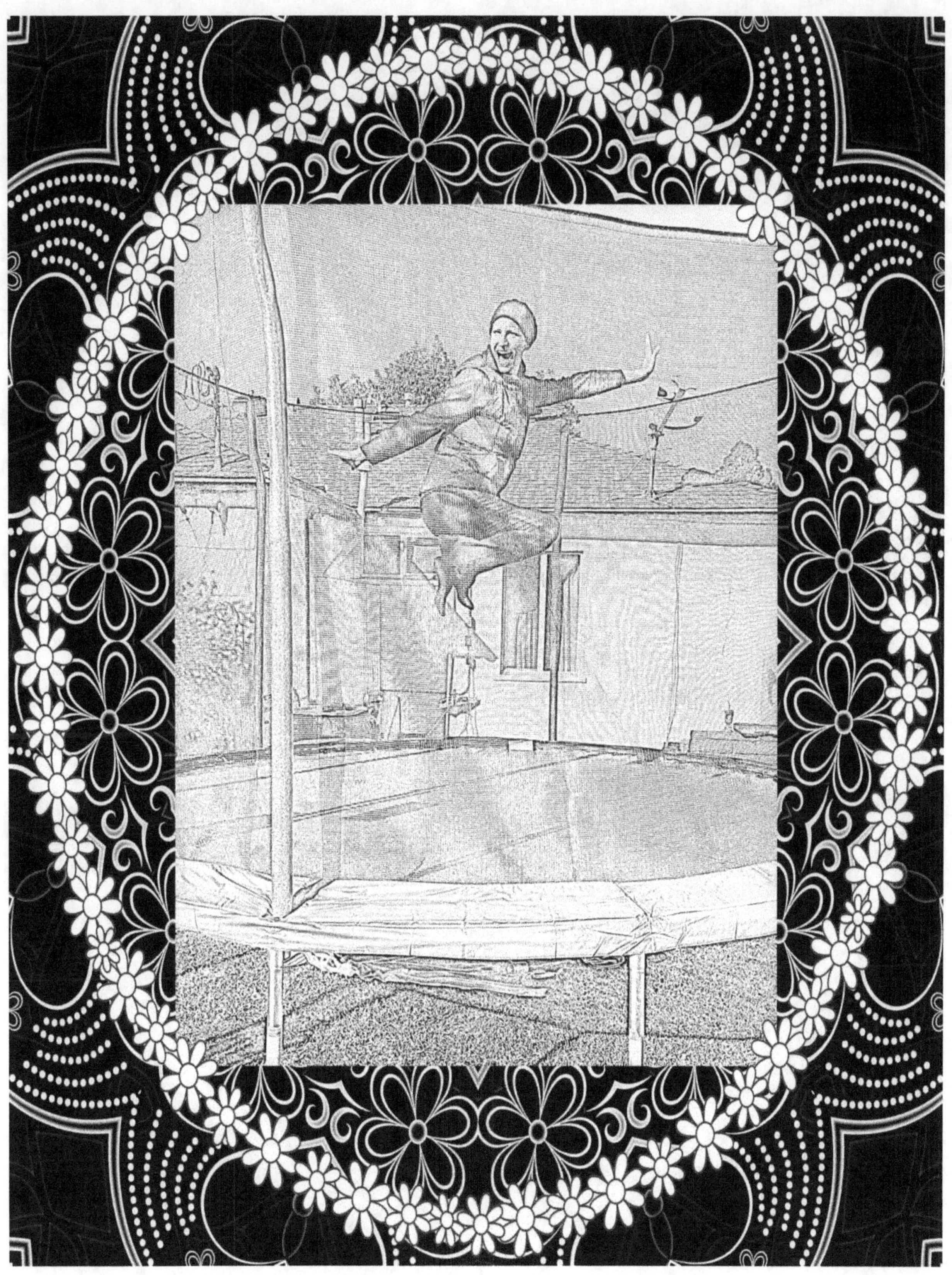

FightLikeaGrownAssWoman.com

FightLikeaGrownAssWoman.com

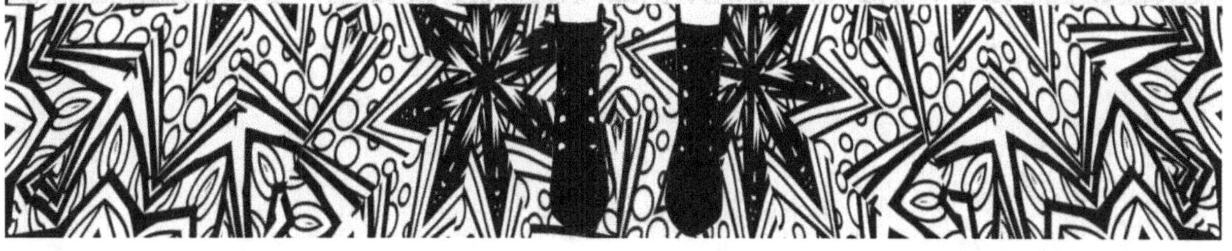

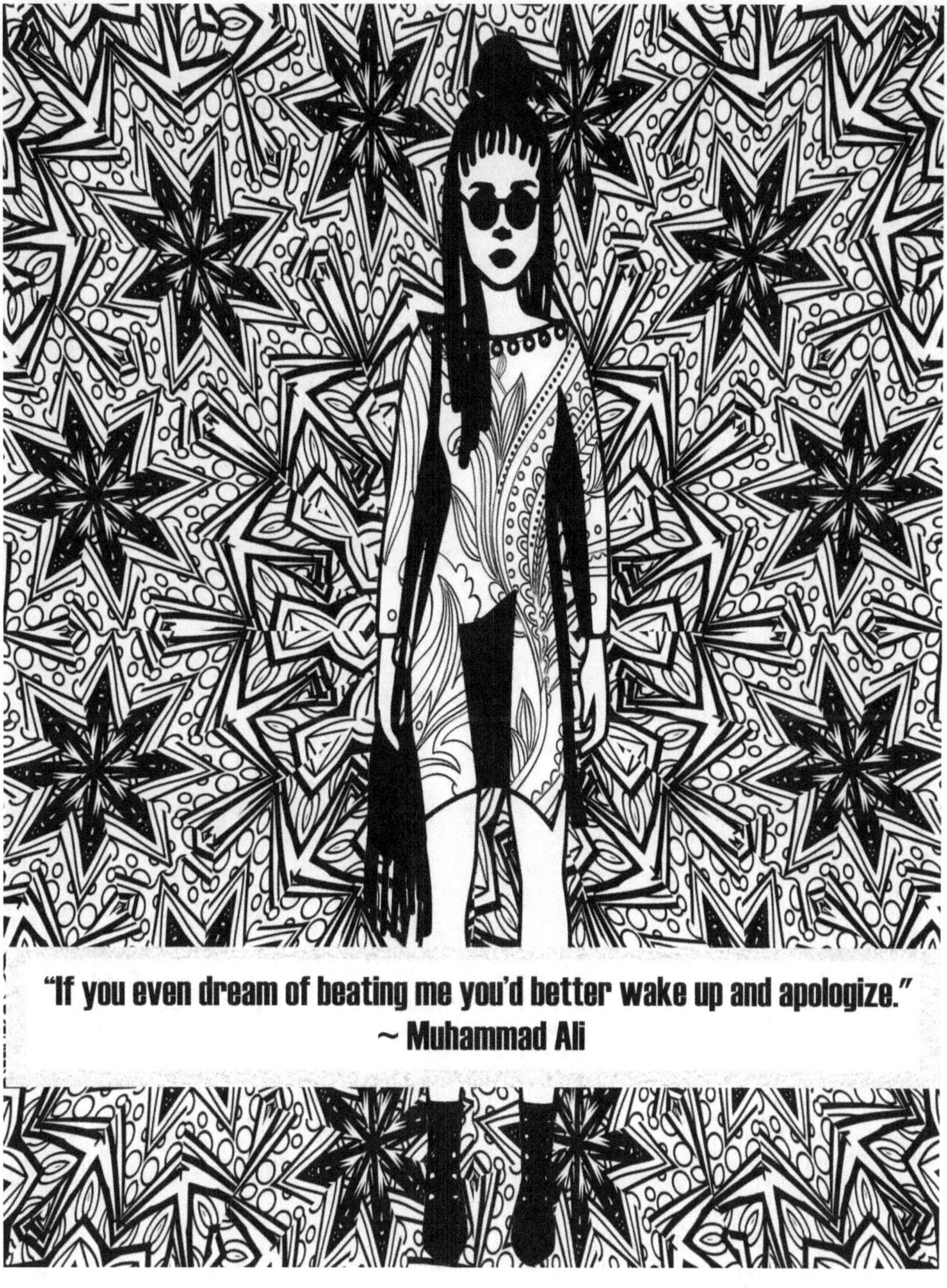

FightLikeaGrownAssWoman.com

FightLikeaGrownAssWoman.com

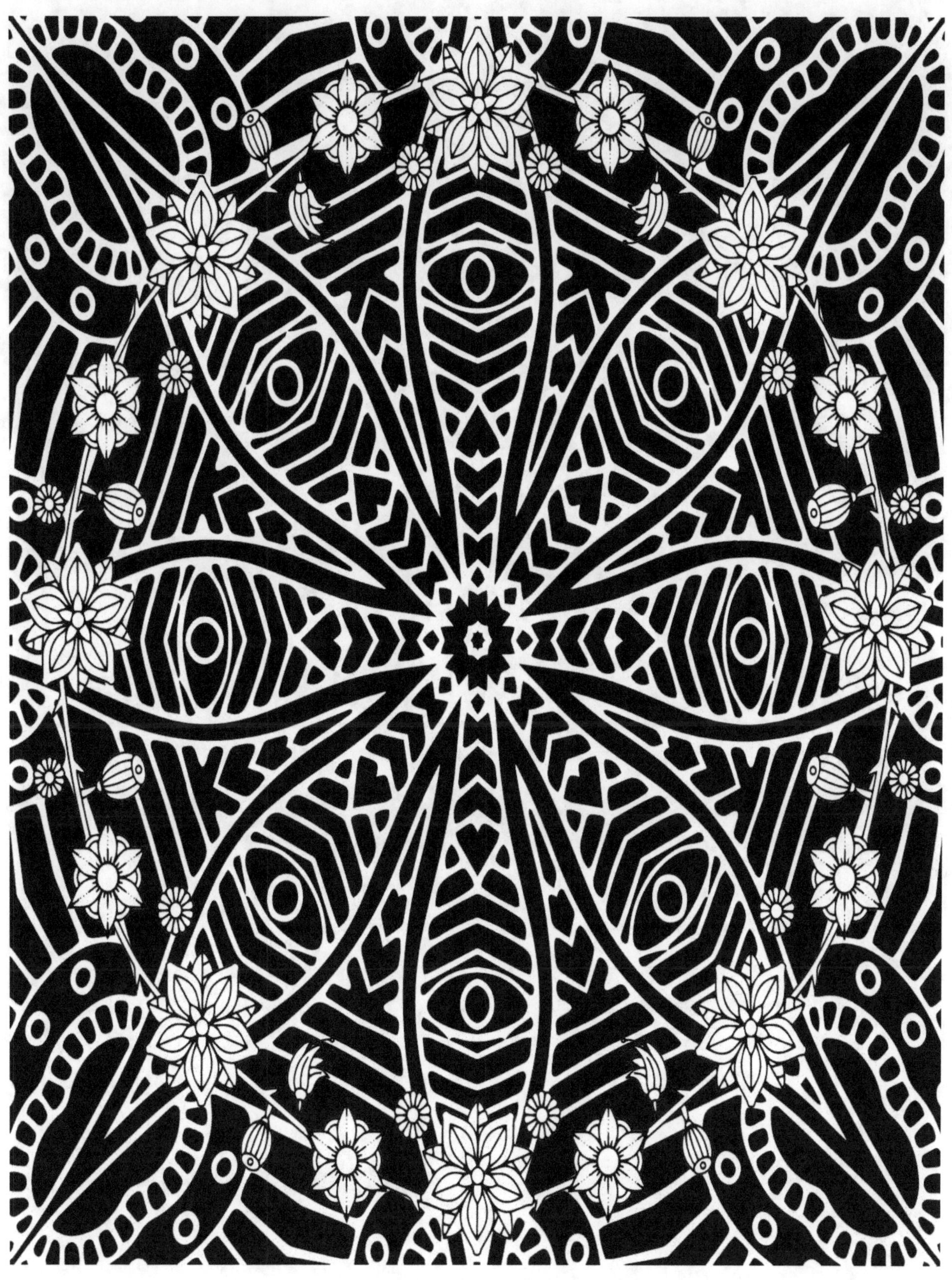

FightLikeaGrownAssWoman.com

FightLikeaGrownAssWoman.com

FightLikeaGrownAssWoman.com

FightLikeaGrownAssWoman.com

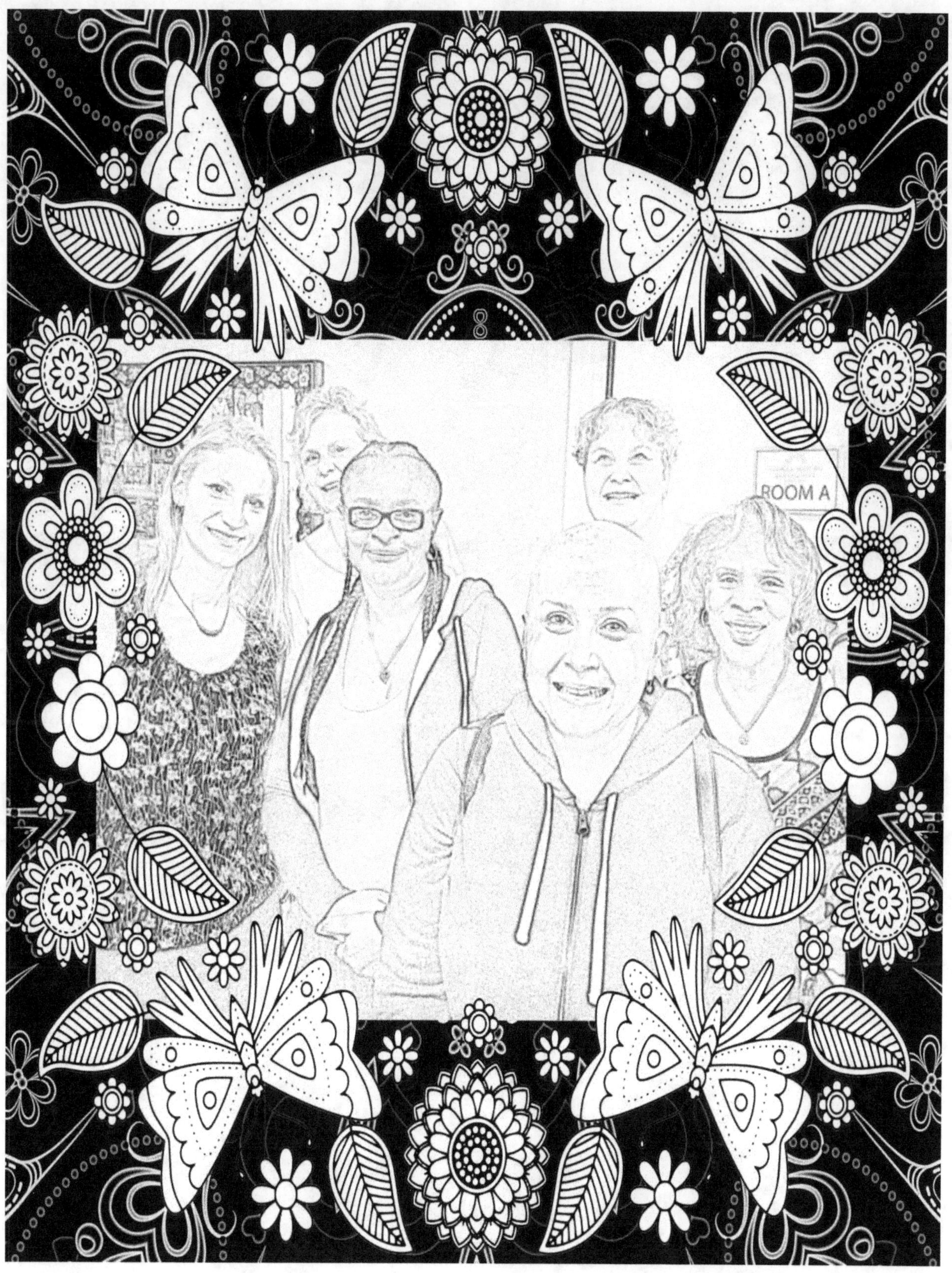

ROOM A

FightLikeaGrownAssWoman.com

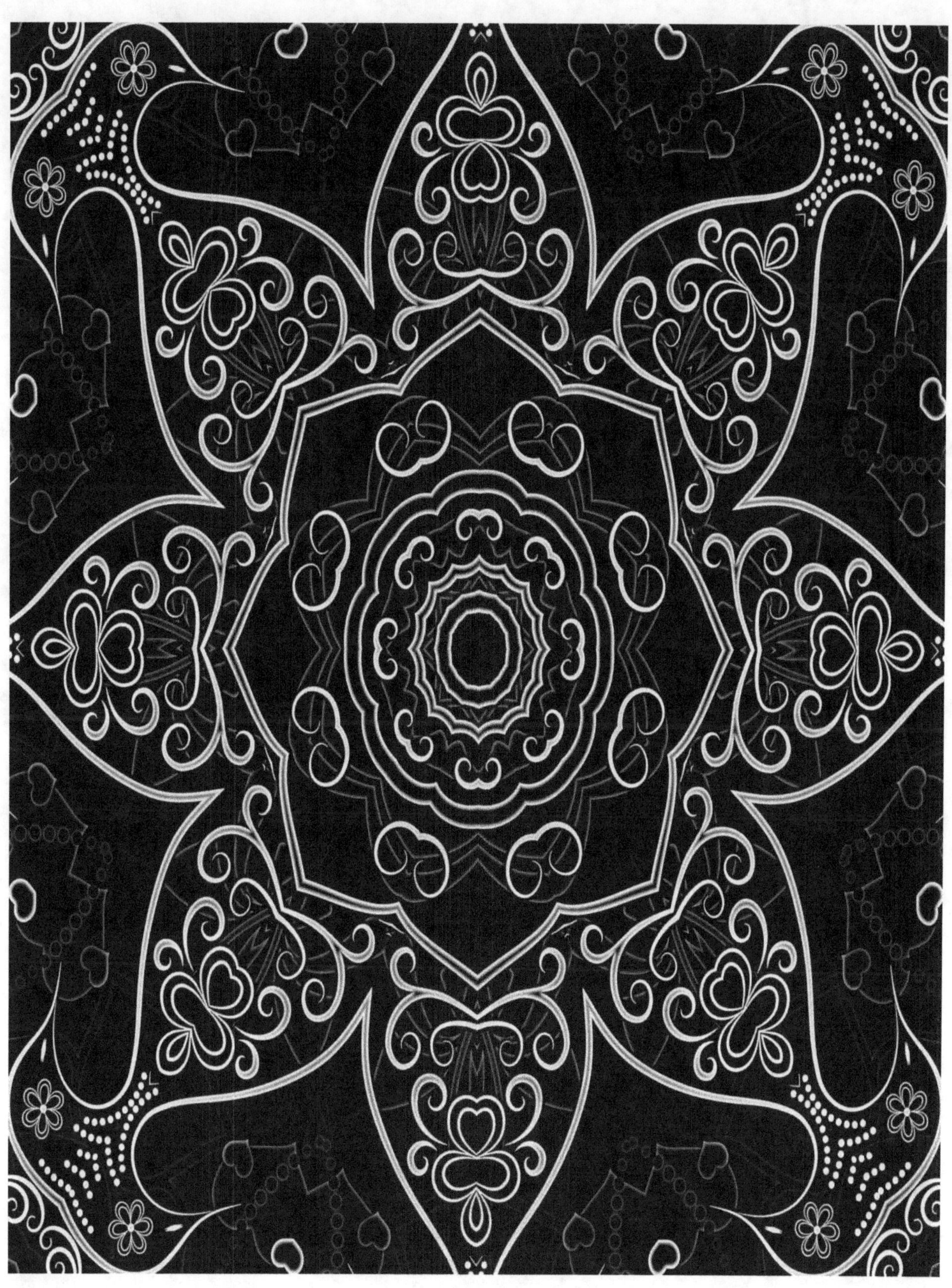

FightLikeaGrownAssWoman.com

FightLikeaGrownAssWoman.com

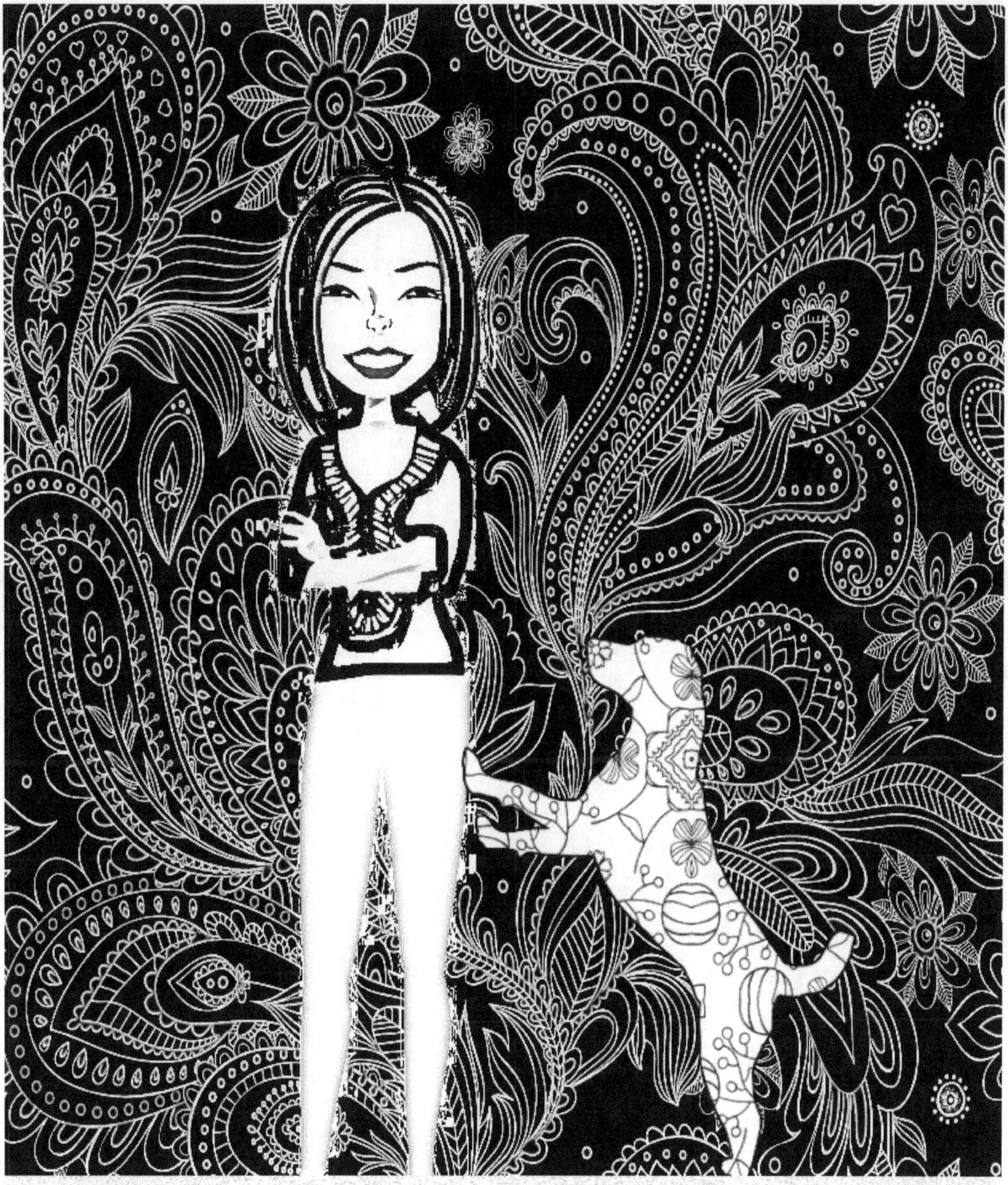

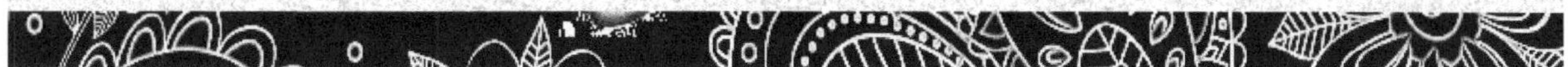

"A lot of people are afraid to say what they want. That's why they don't get what they want."
~ Madonna

FightLikeaGrownAssWoman.com

FightLikeaGrownAssWoman.com

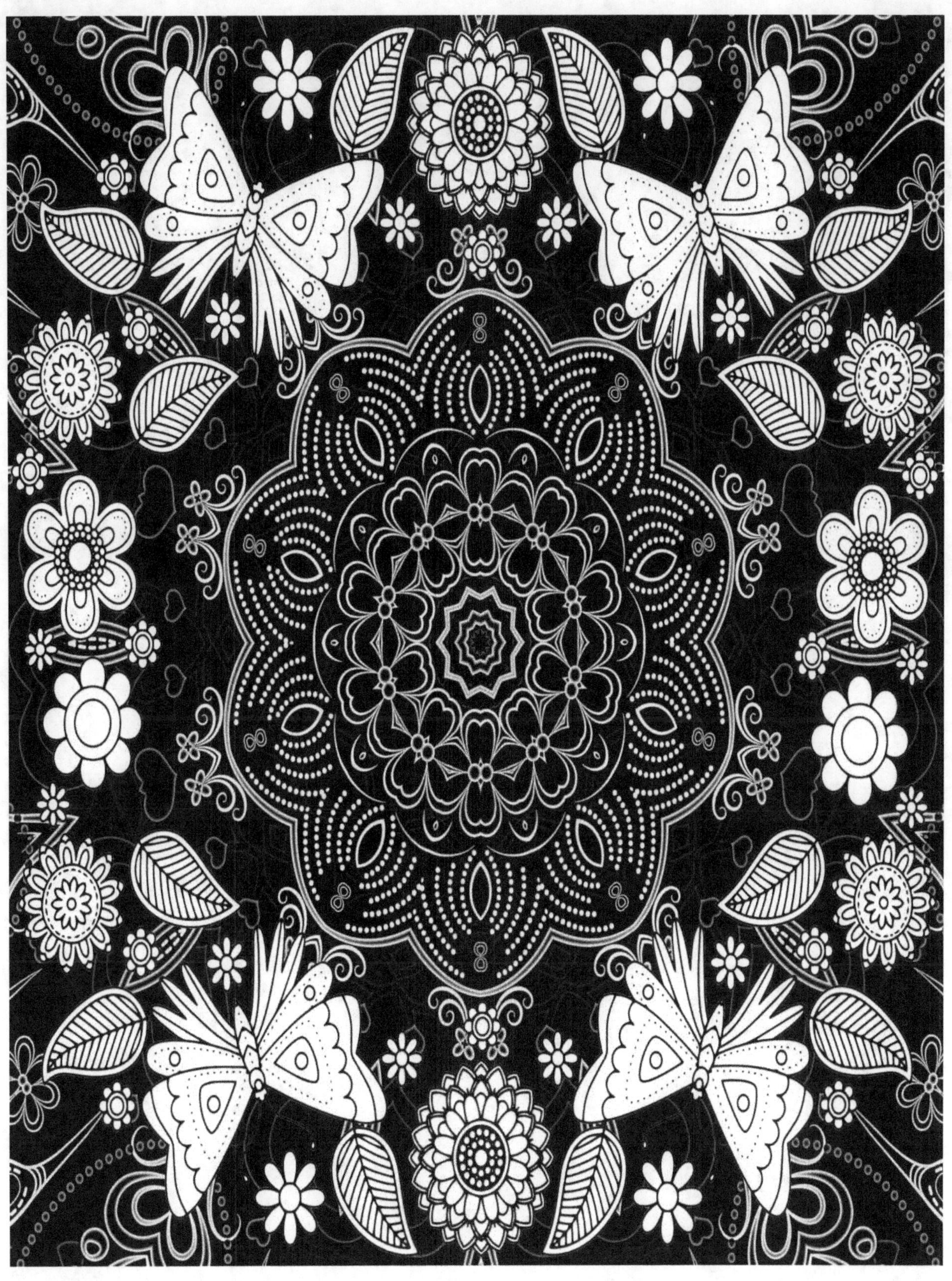

FightLikeaGrownAssWoman.com

FightLikeaGrownAssWoman.com

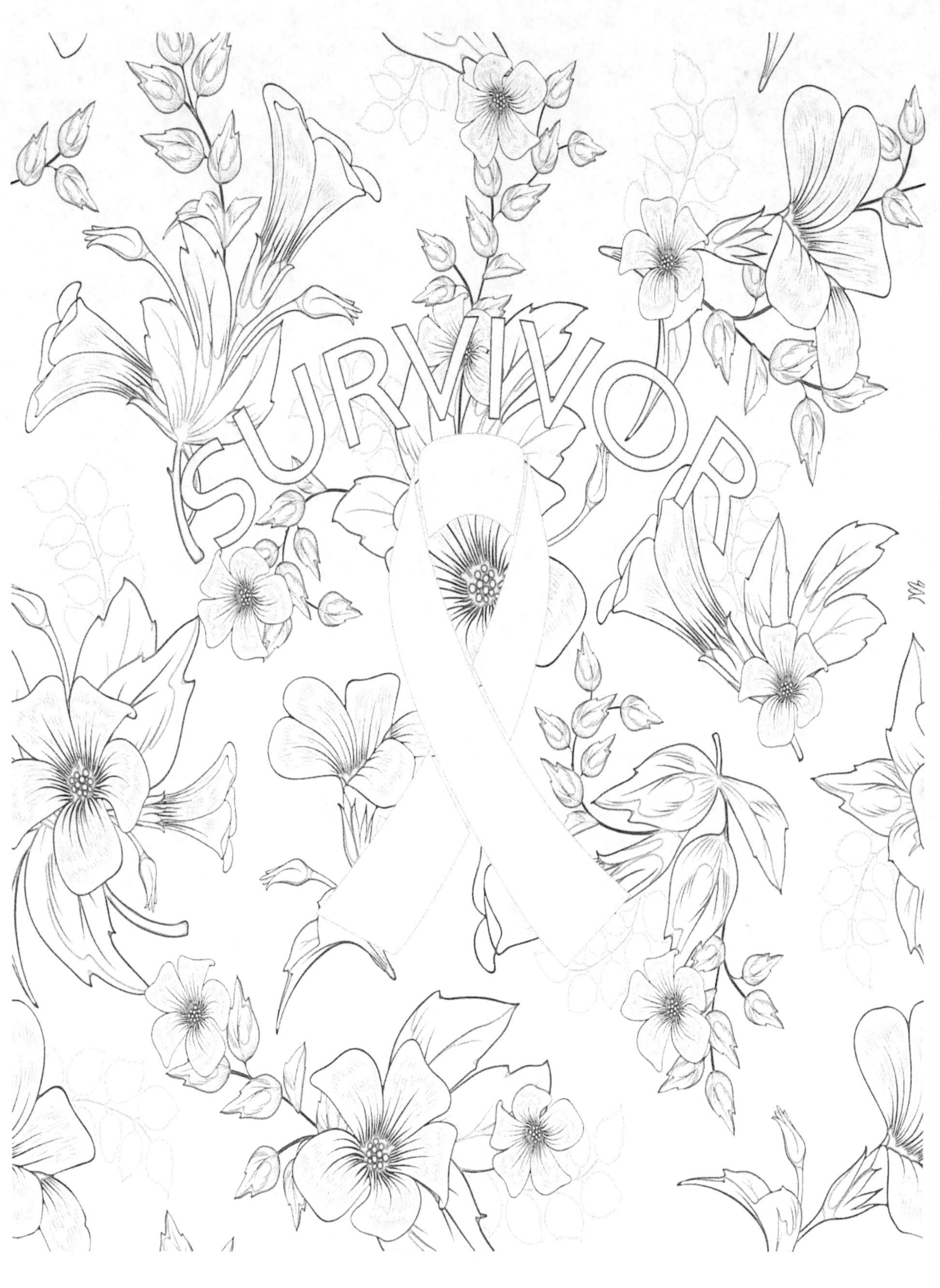

FightLikeaGrownAssWoman.com

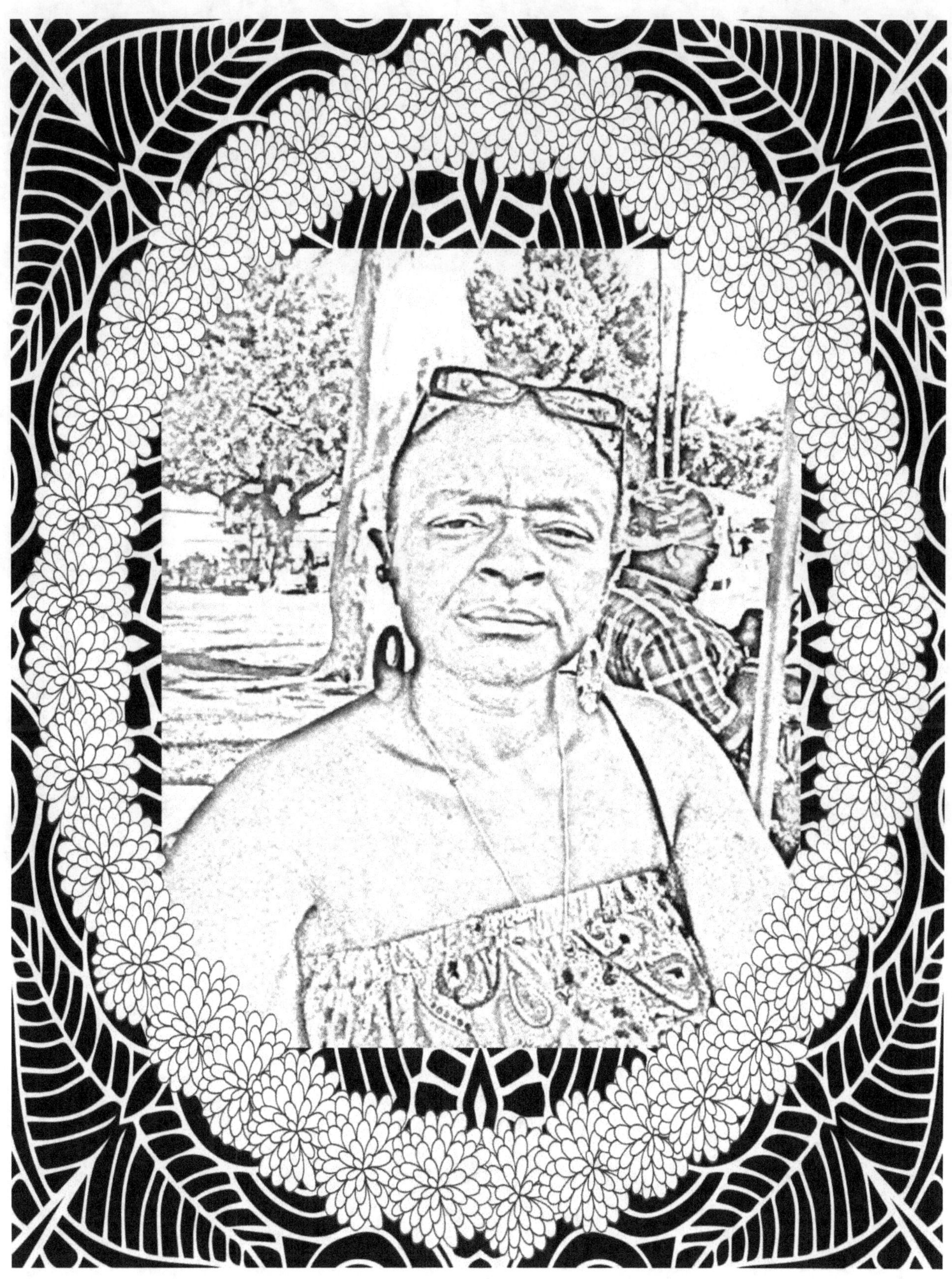

FightLikeaGrownAssWoman.com

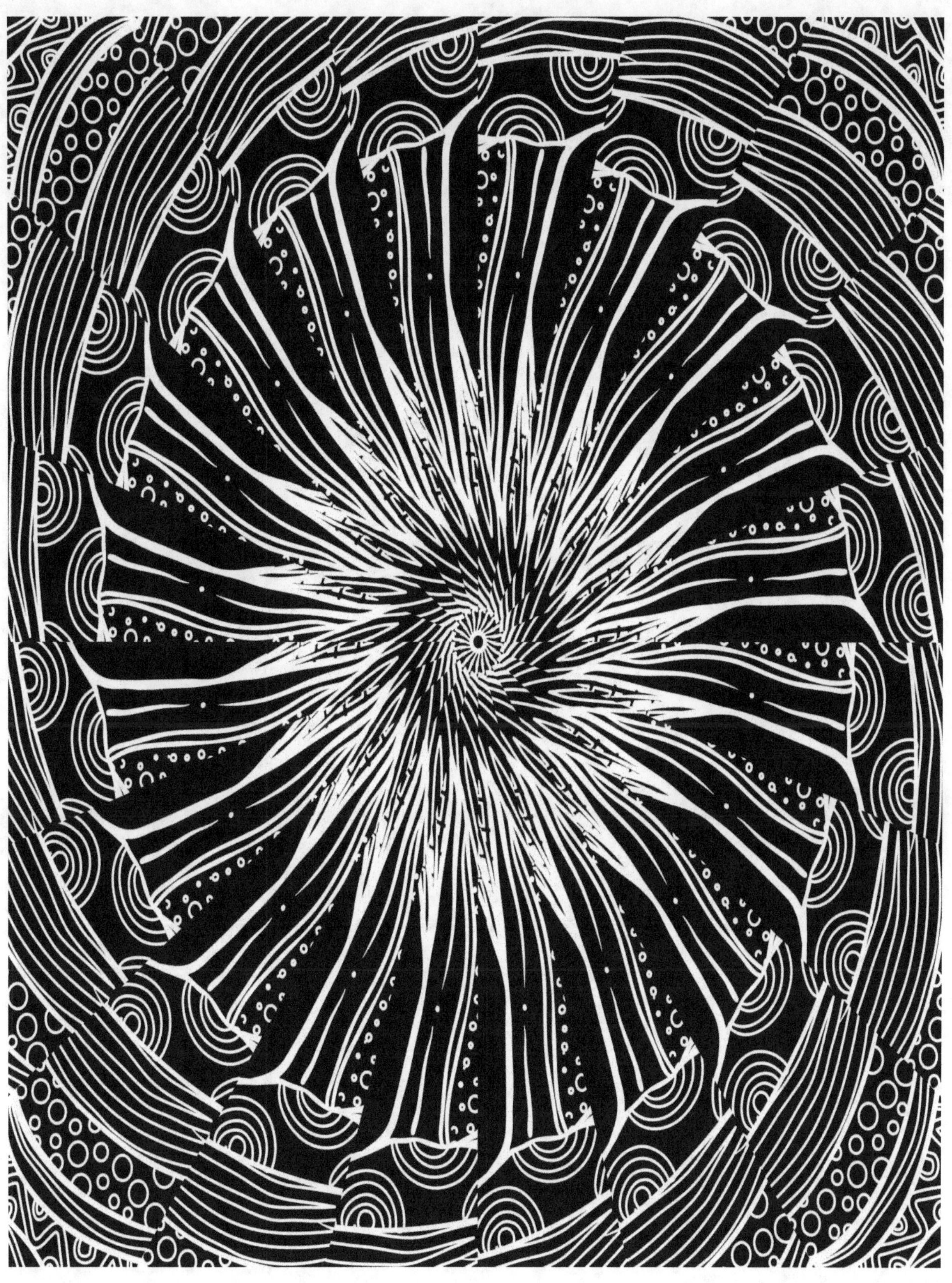

FightLikeaGrownAssWoman.com

FightLikeaGrownAssWoman.com

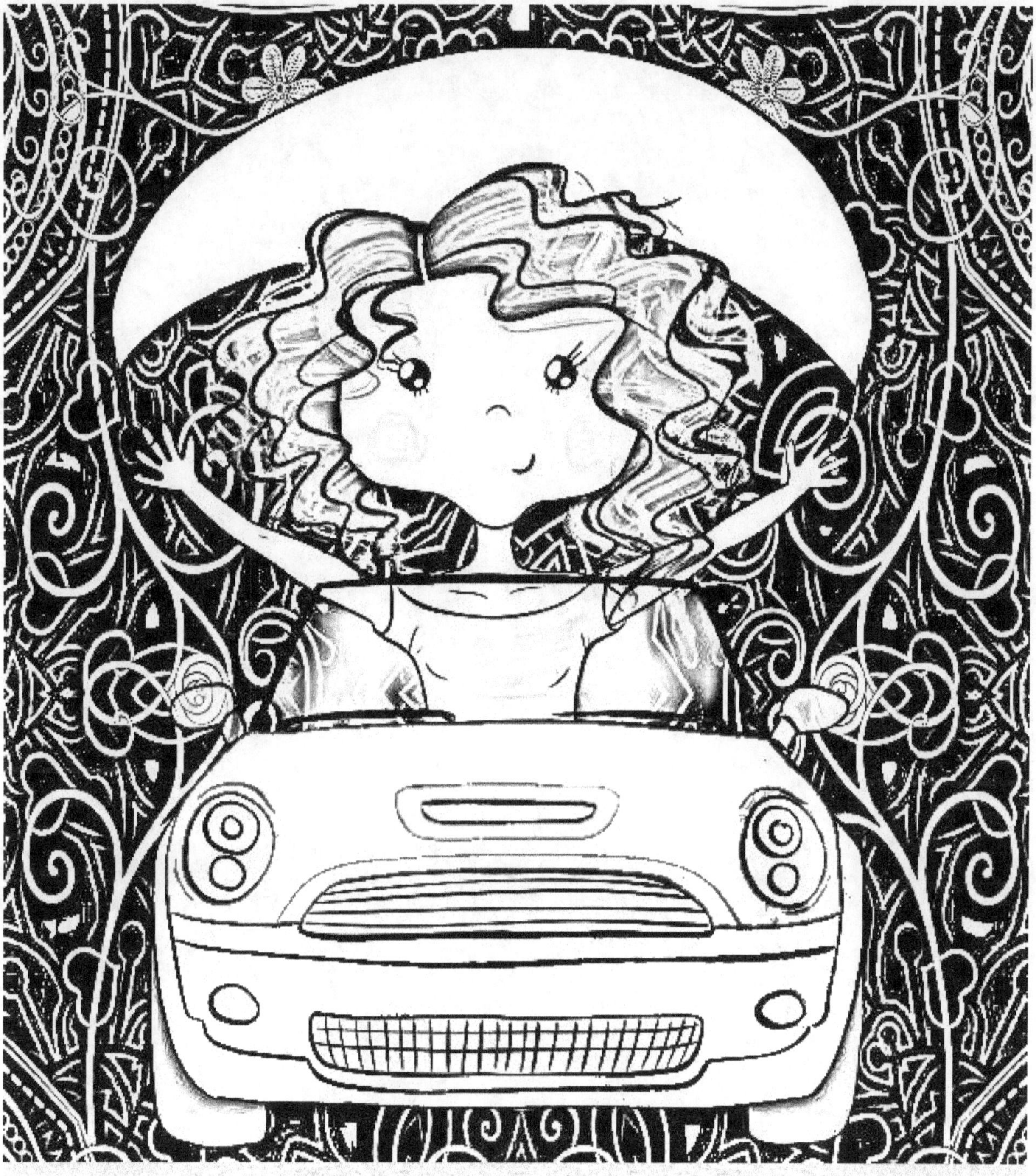

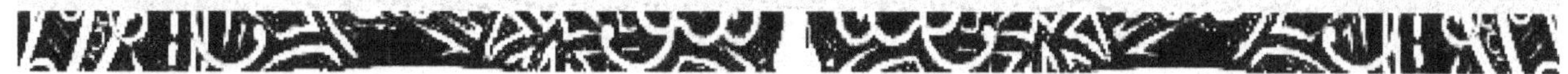

"One day your life will flash before your eyes. Make sure it's worth watching."
~ Unkown

FightLikeaGrownAssWoman.com

FightLikeaGrownAssWoman.com

FightLikeaGrownAssWoman.com

FightLikeaGrownAssWoman.com

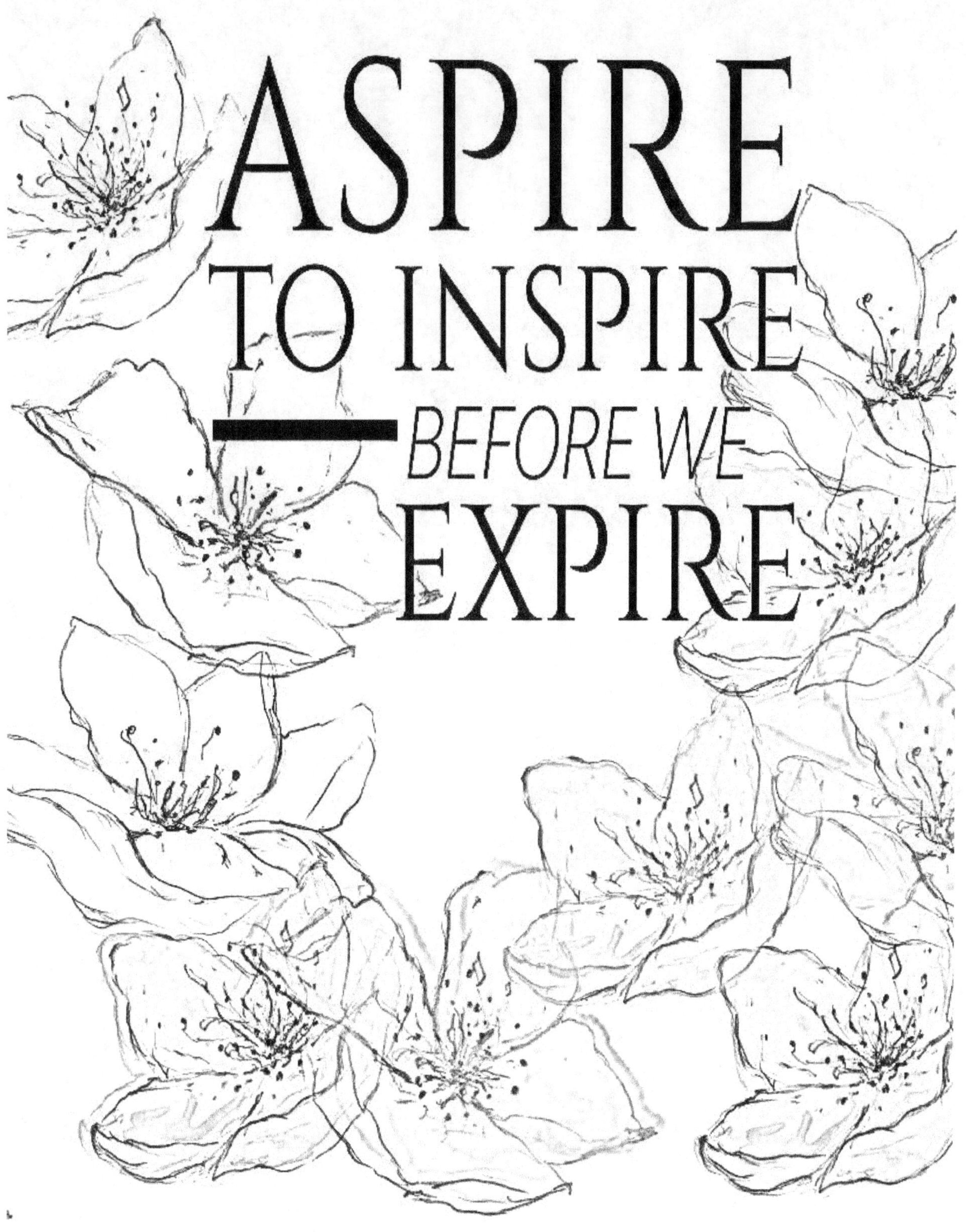

ASPIRE
TO INSPIRE
BEFORE WE
EXPIRE

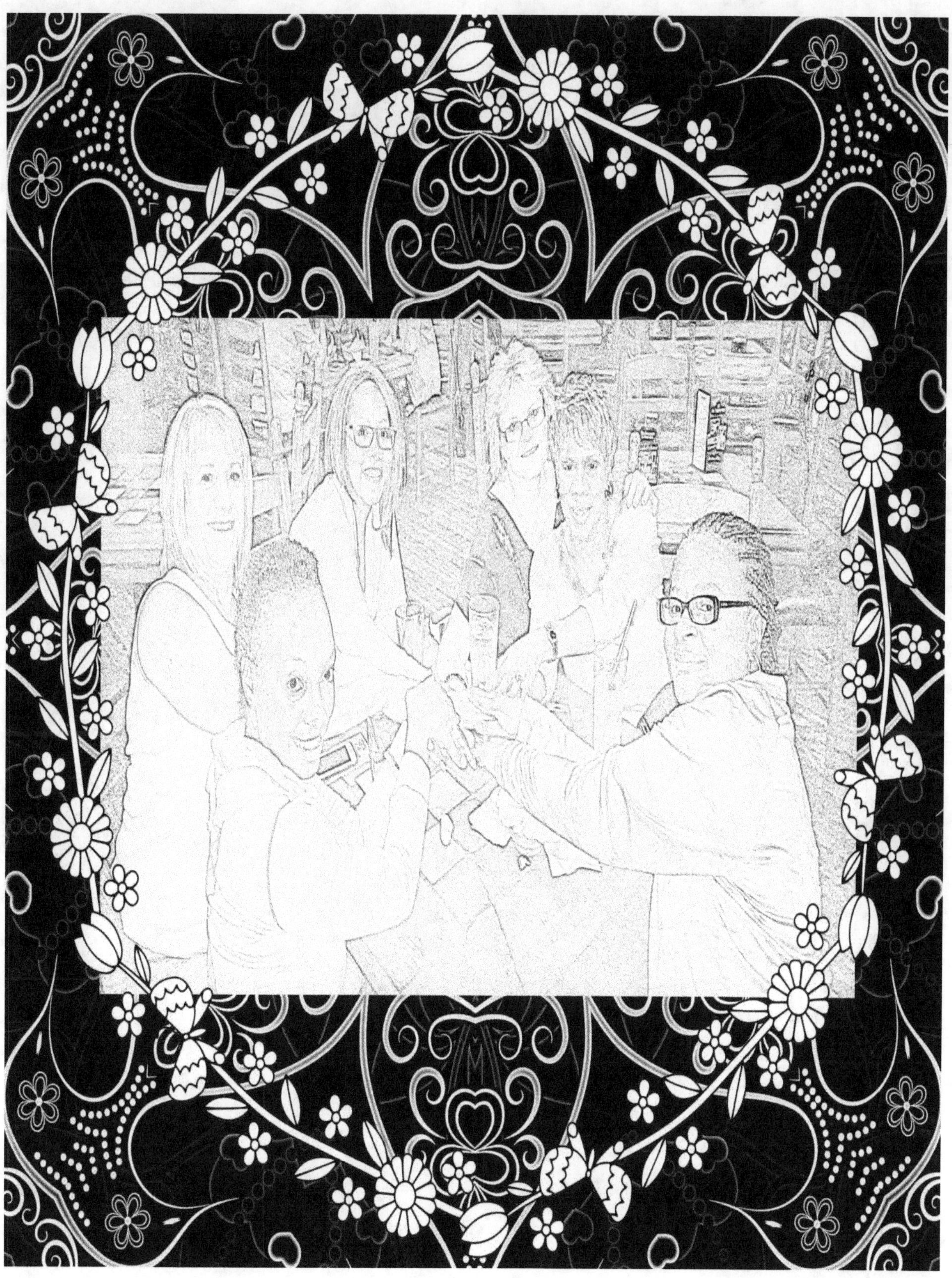

FightLikeaGrownAssWoman.com

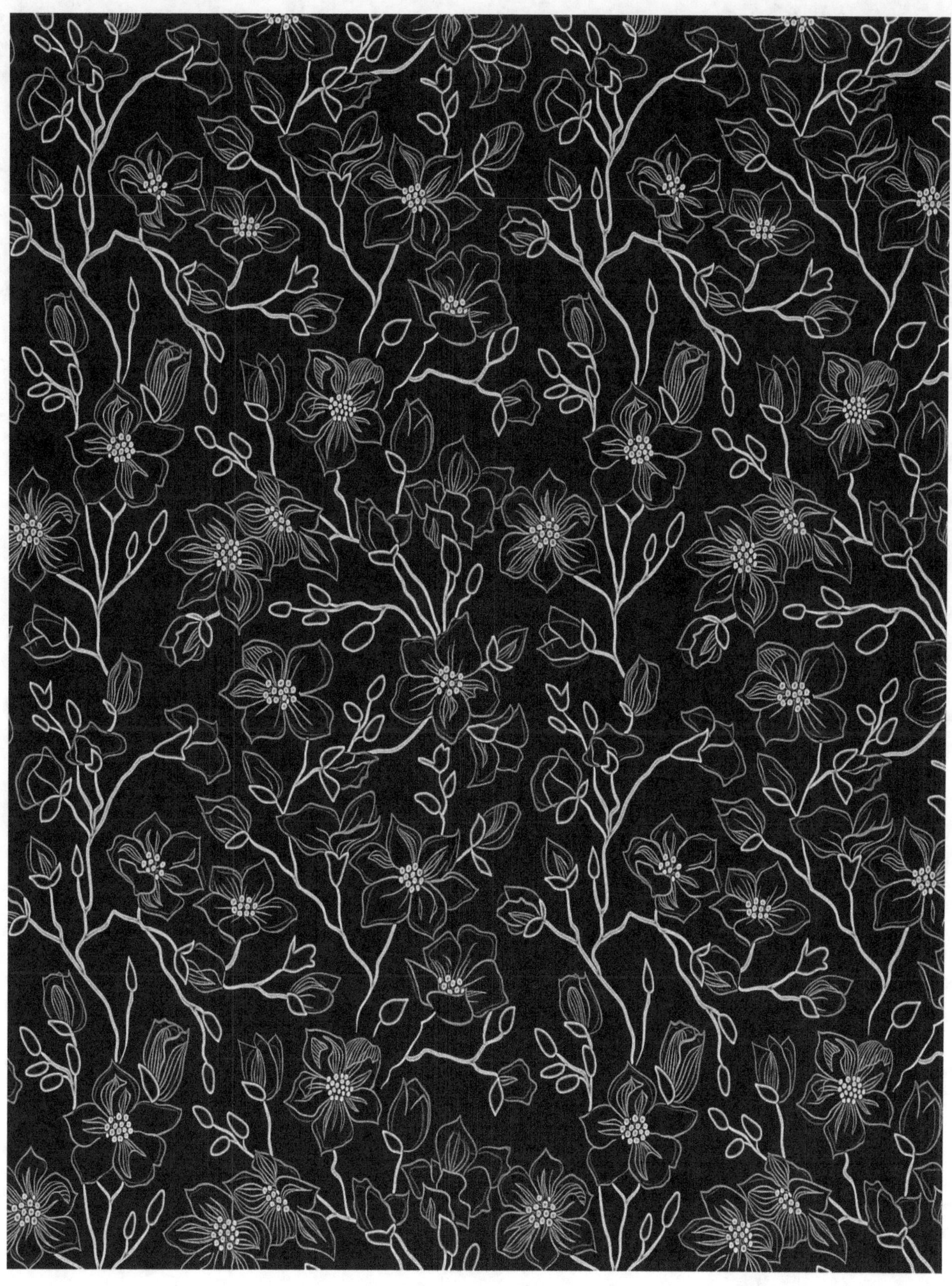

FightLikeaGrownAssWoman.com

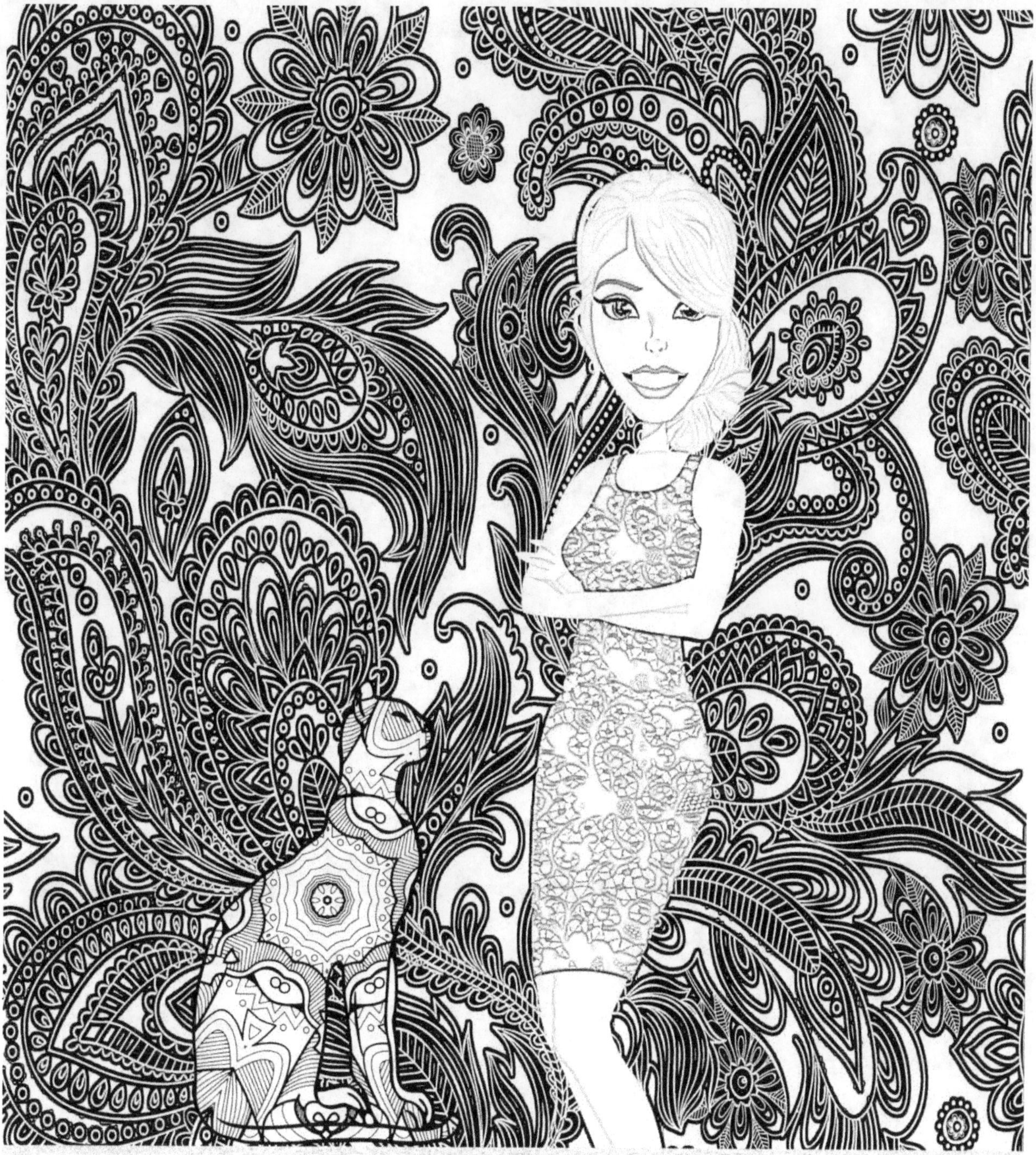

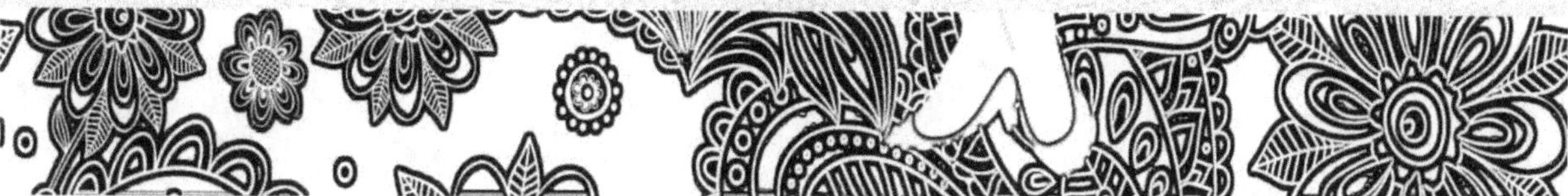

"If you wanna fly, you got to give up the shit that weighs you down."
~ Toni Morrison

FightLikeaGrownAssWoman.com

FightLikeaGrownAssWoman.com

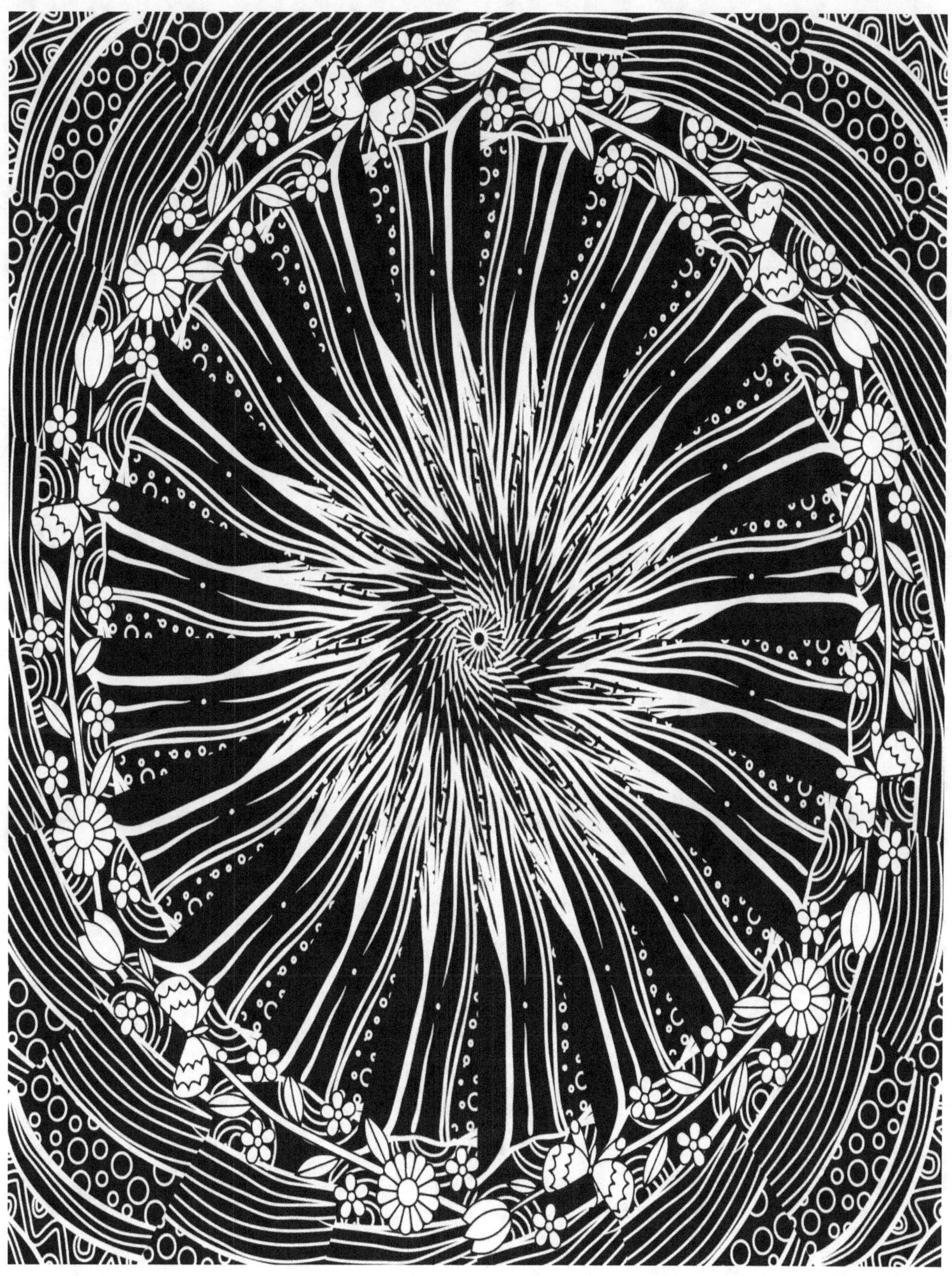

FightLikeaGrownAssWoman.com

FightLikeaGrownAssWoman.com

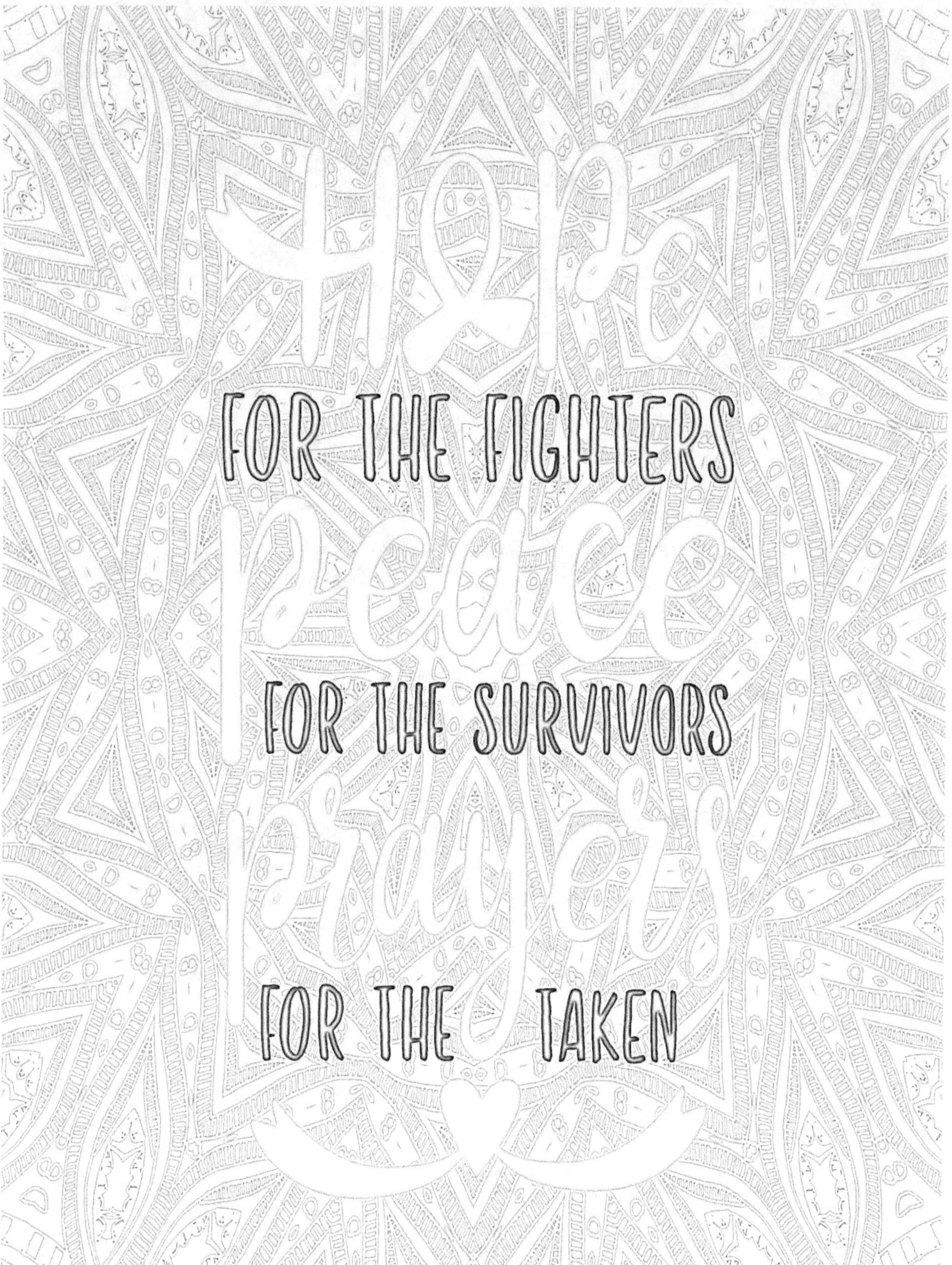

Hope
FOR THE FIGHTERS
peace
FOR THE SURVIVORS
prayers
FOR THE   TAKEN

FightLikeaGrownAssWoman.com

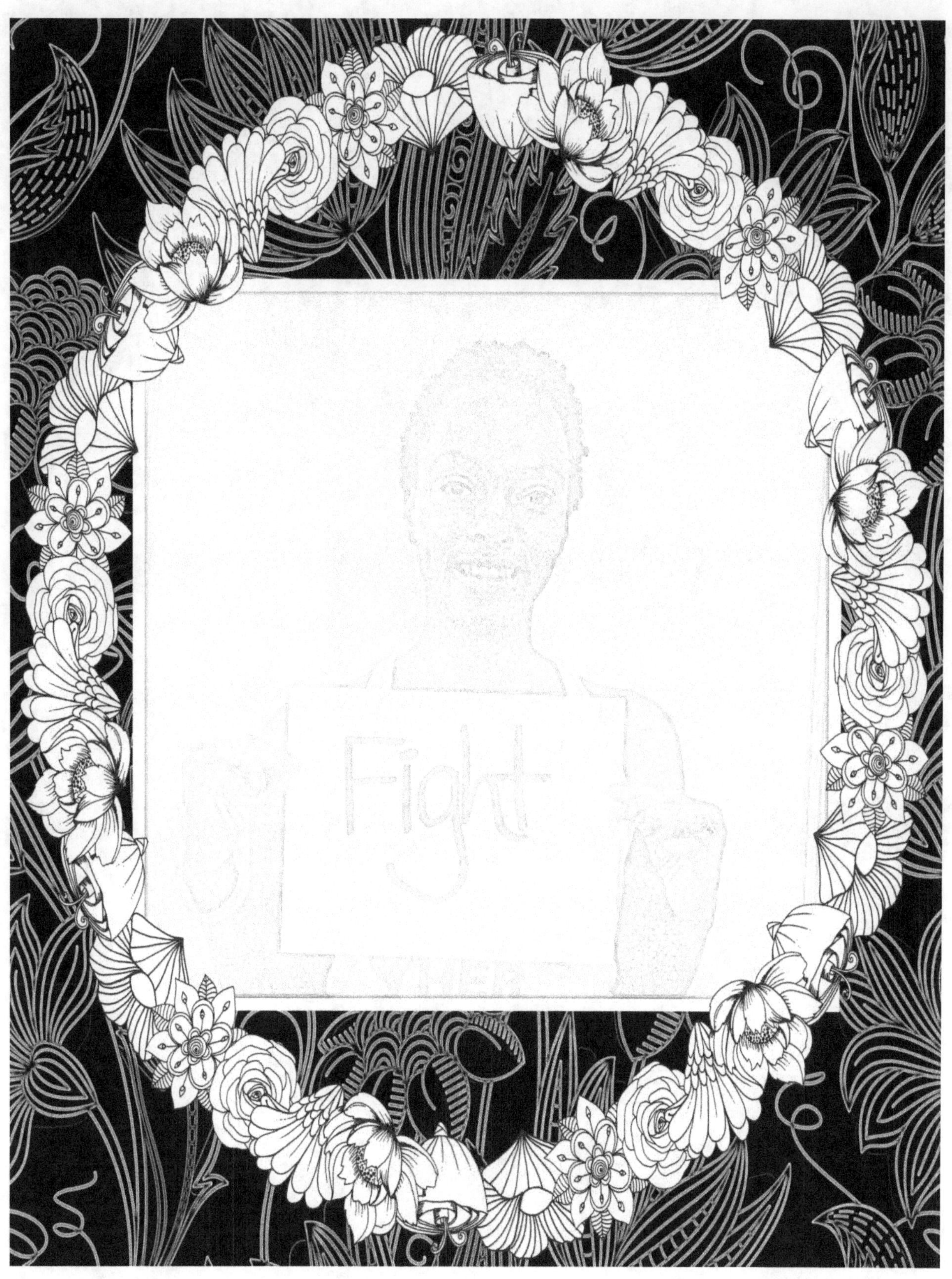

Fight

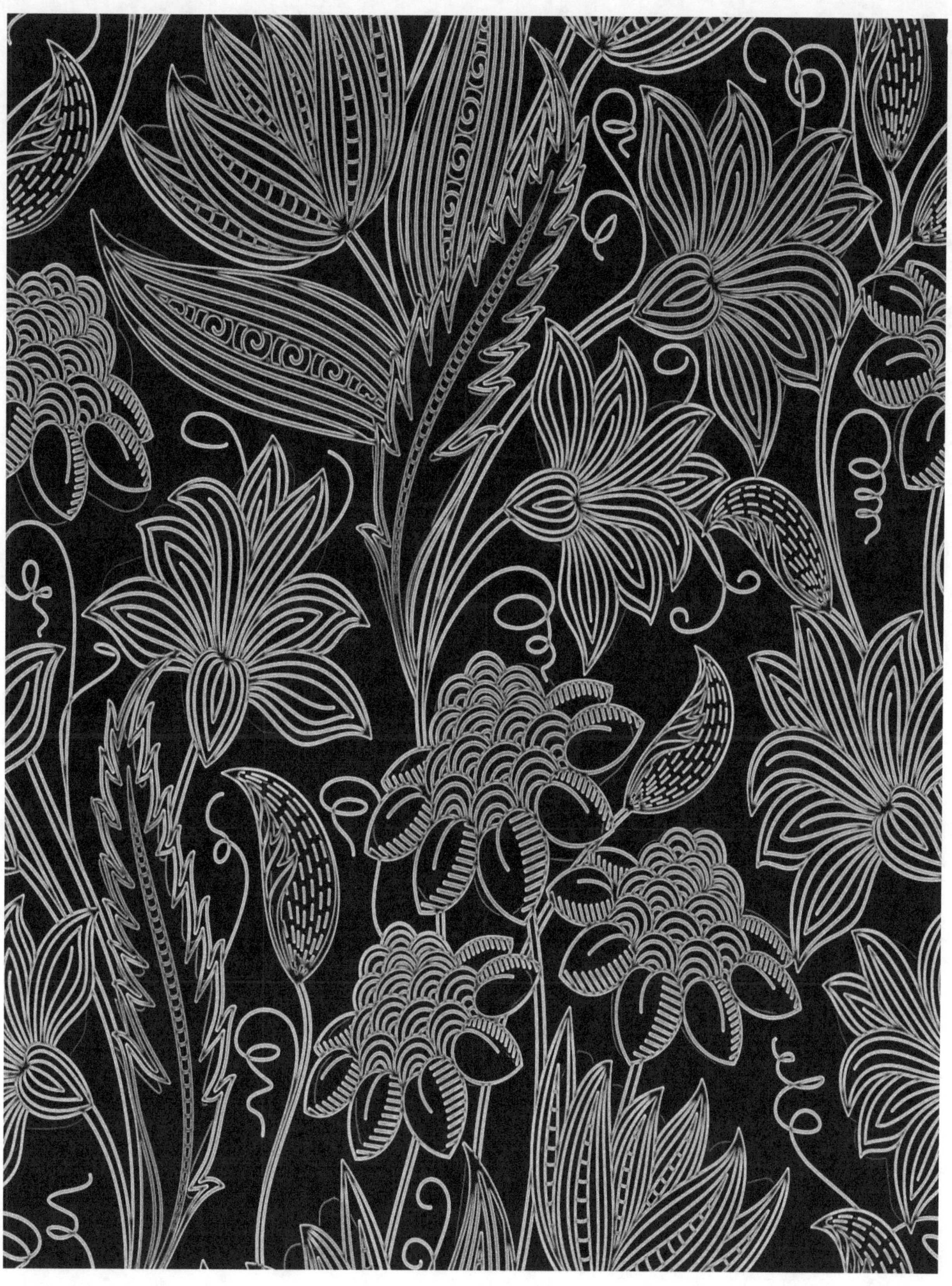

FightLikeaGrownAssWoman.com

FightLikeaGrownAssWoman.com

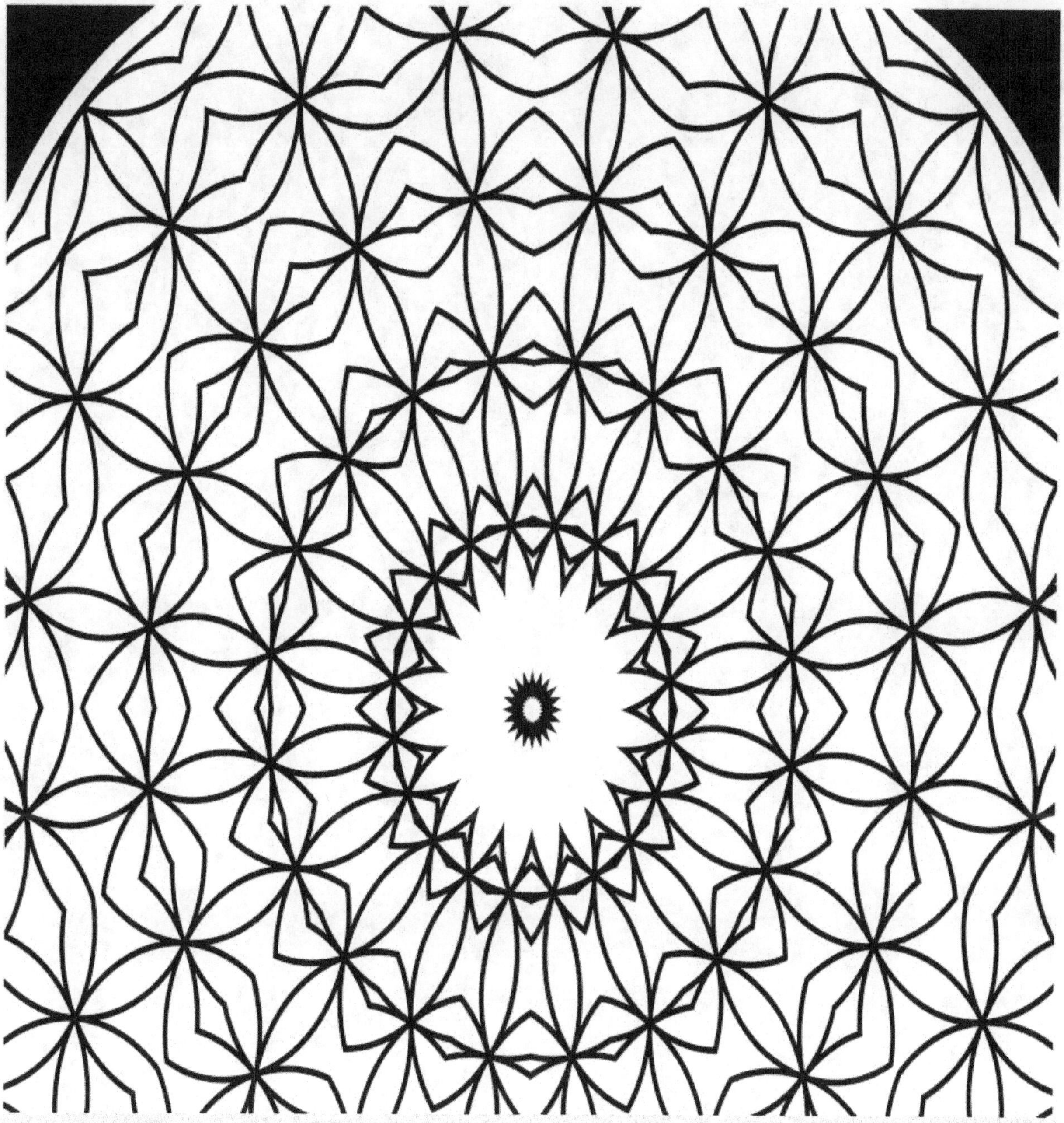

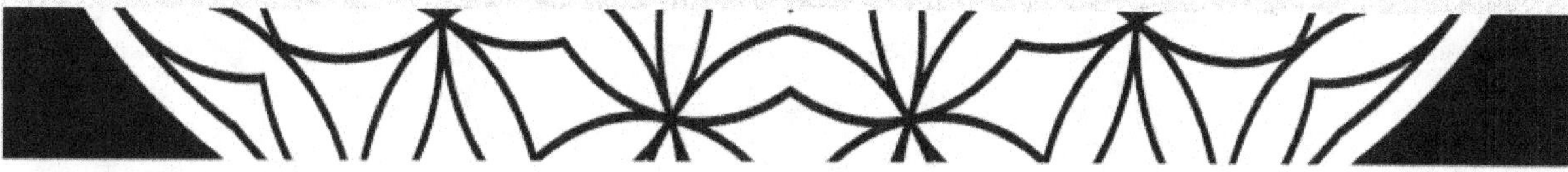

"Begin doing what you want to do now. We have only this moment,
sparkling like a star in our hand, and melting like a snowflake."
~~Marie Ray

FightLikeaGrownAssWoman.com

FightLikeaGrownAssWoman.com

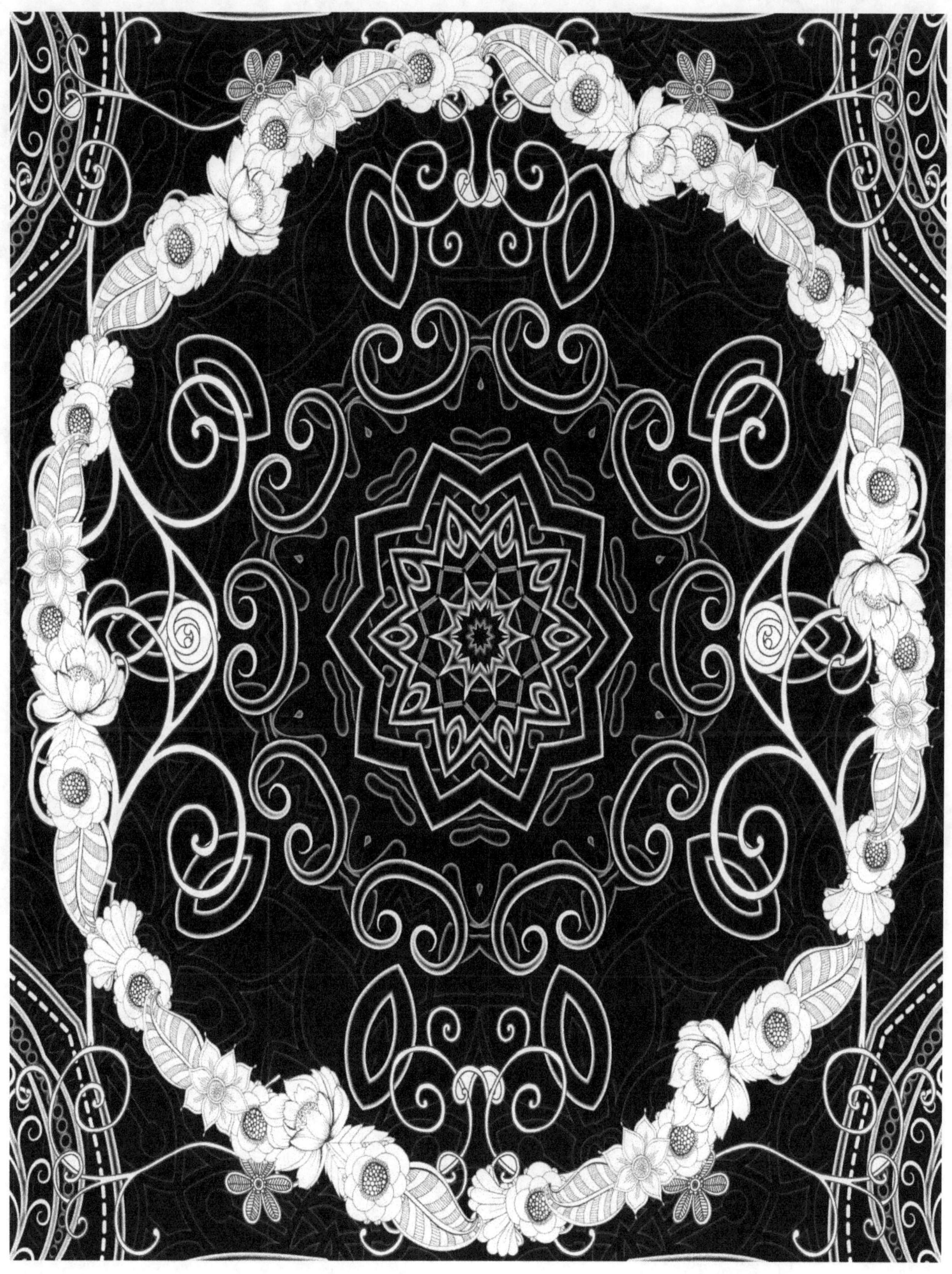

FightLikeaGrownAssWoman.com

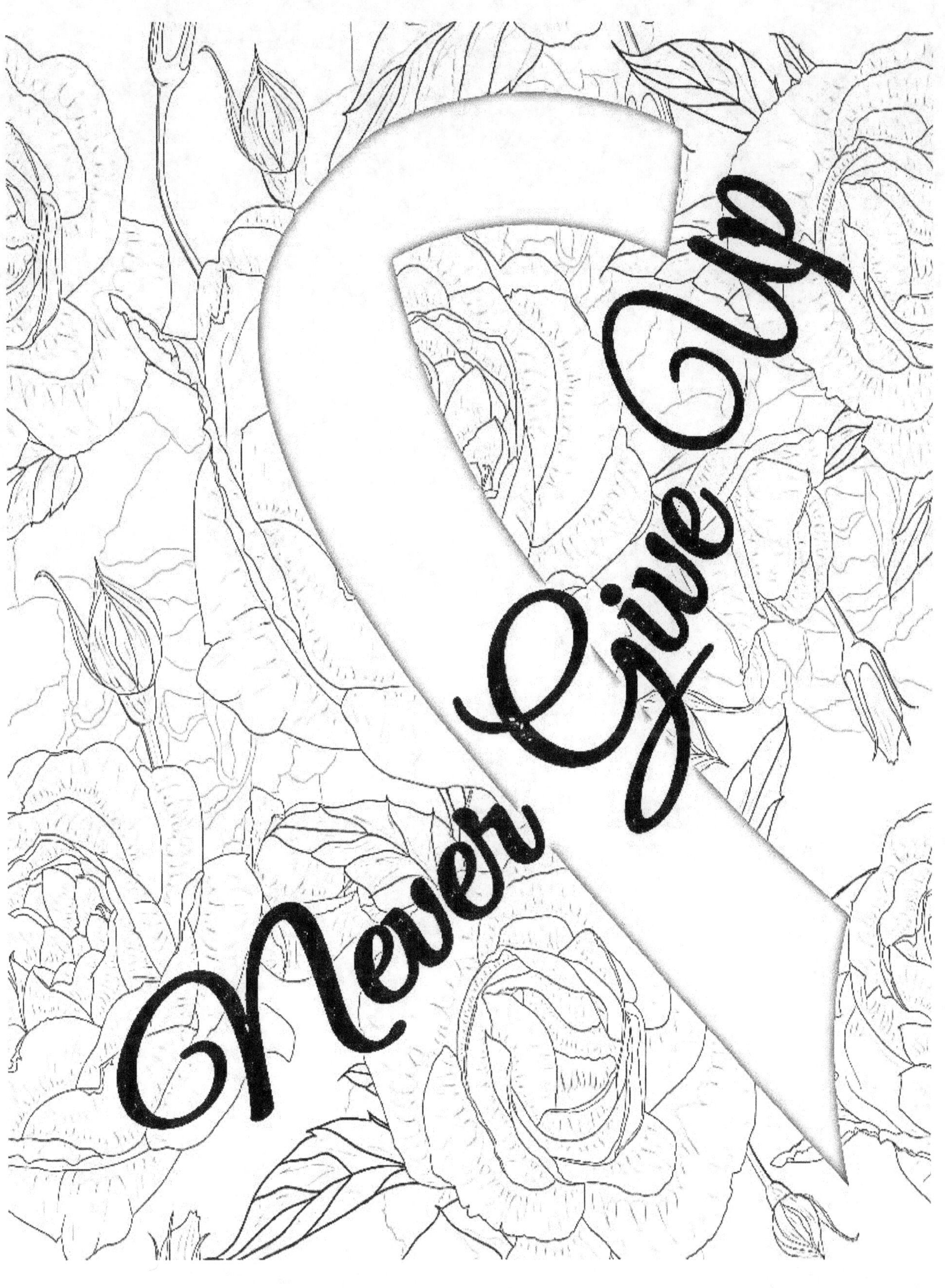

FightLikeaGrownAssWoman.com

FightLikeaGrownAssWoman.com

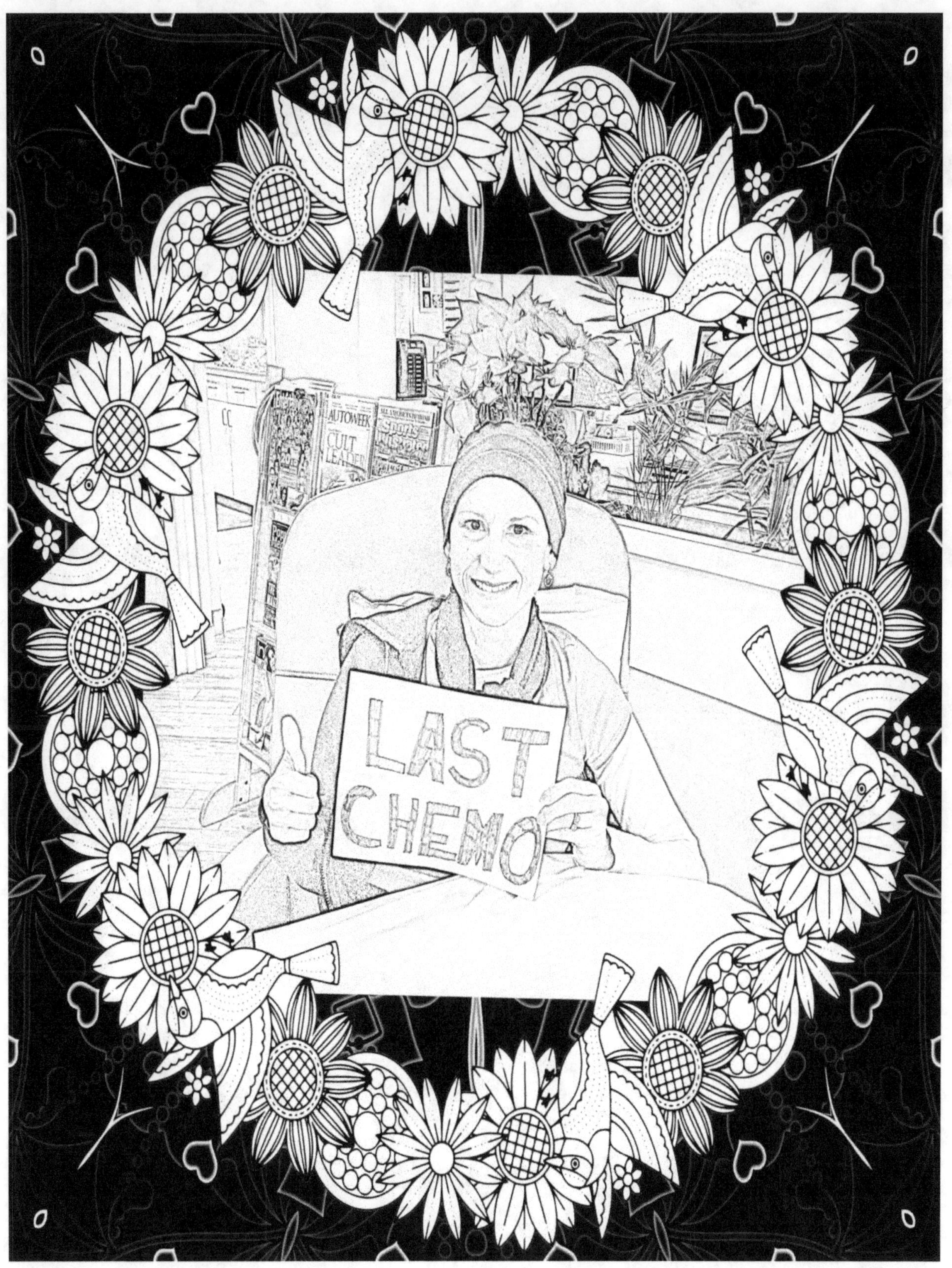

FightLikeaGrownAssWoman.com

FightLikeaGrownAssWoman.com

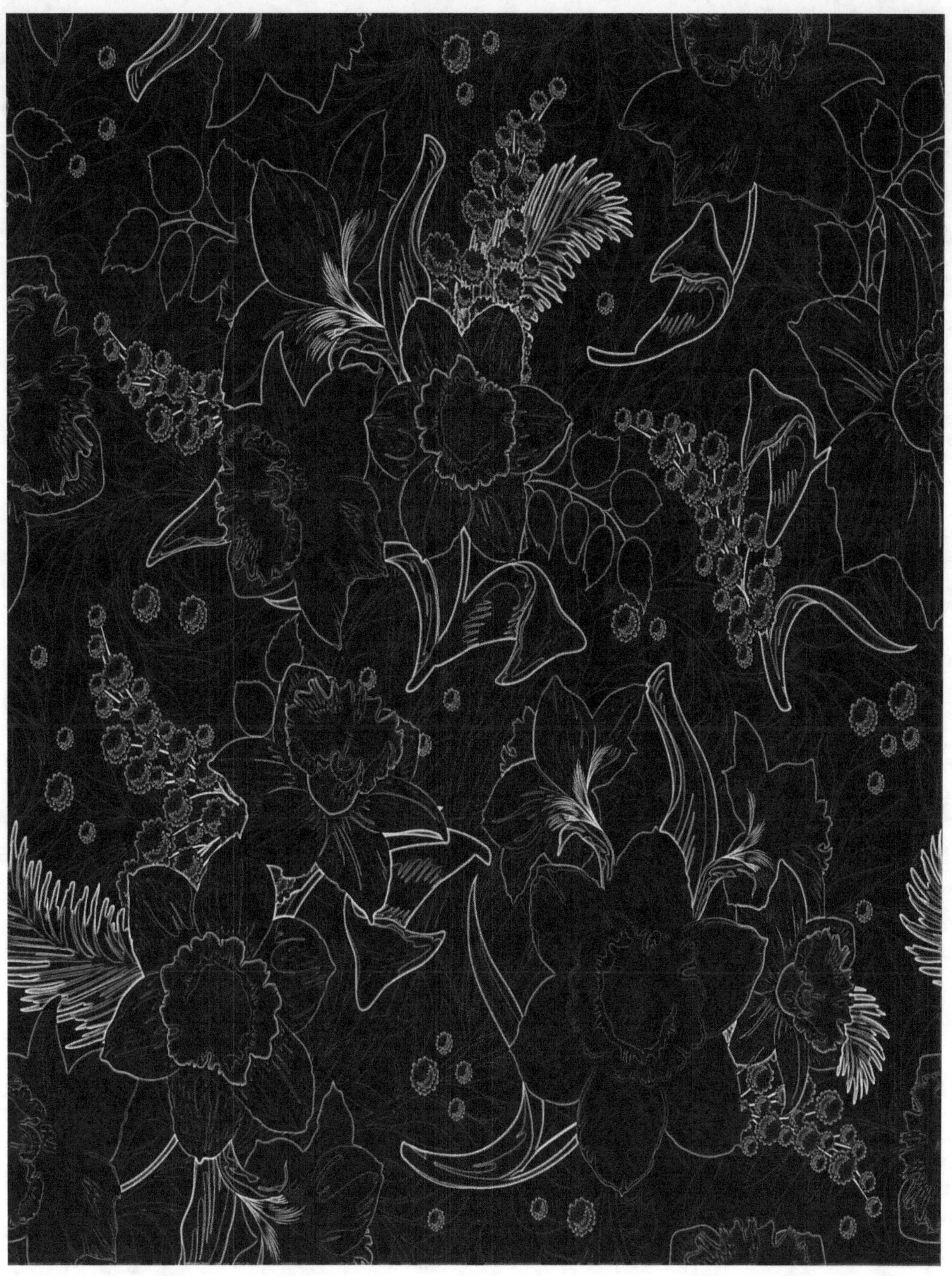

FightLikeaGrownAssWoman.com

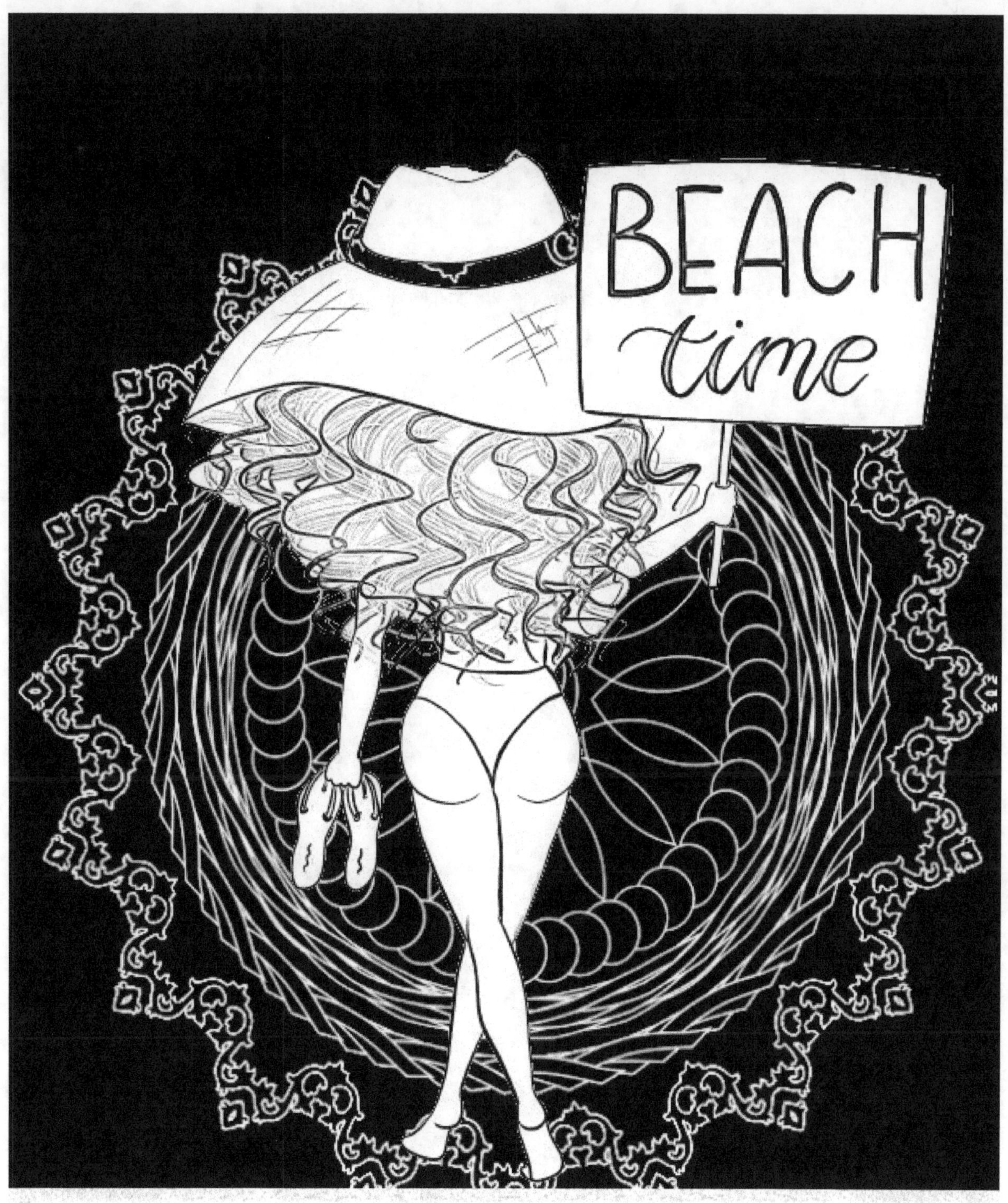

"You live longer once you realize that any time spent being unhappy is wasted. "
~Ruth E. Renkl

FightLikeaGrownAssWoman.com

FightLikeaGrownAssWoman.com

FightLikeaGrownAssWoman.com

FightLikeaGrownAssWoman.com

Giving Up
is simply not an
OPTION

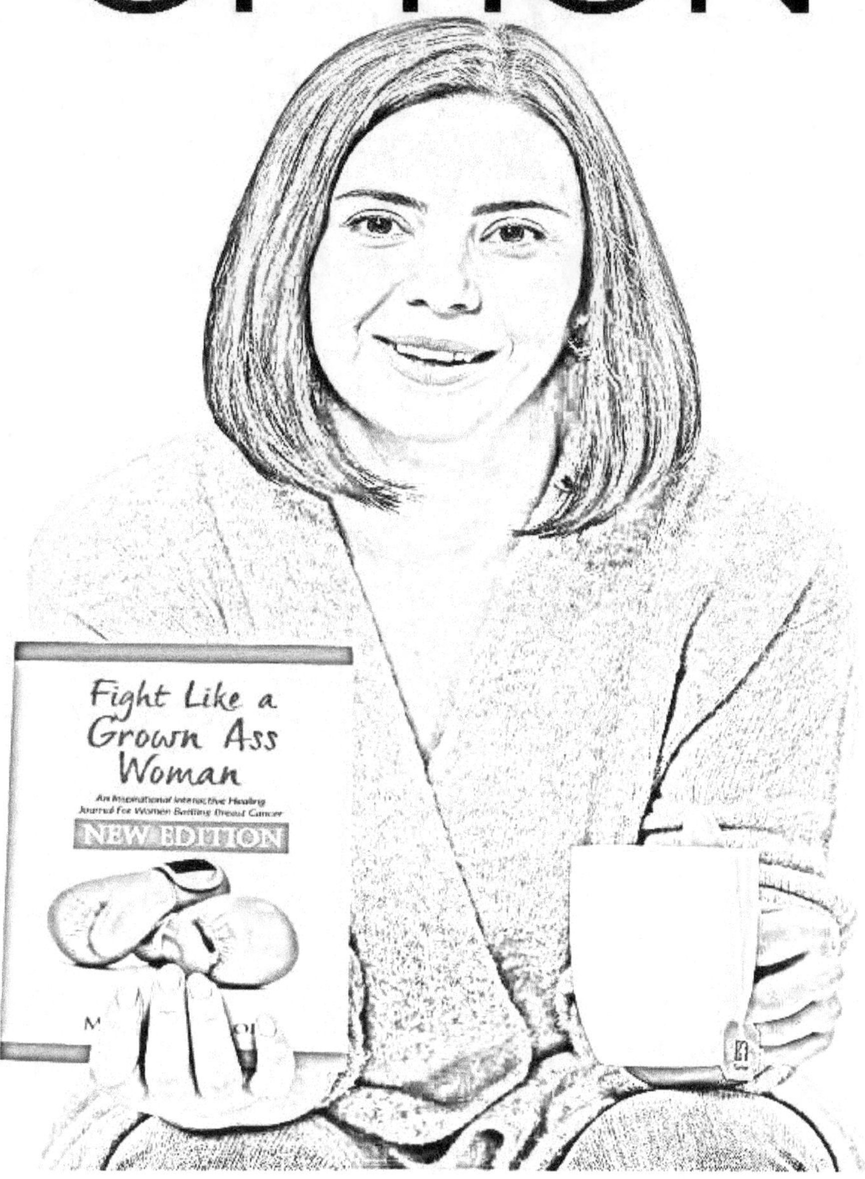

FightLikeaGrownAssWoman.com

FightLikeaGrownAssWoman.com

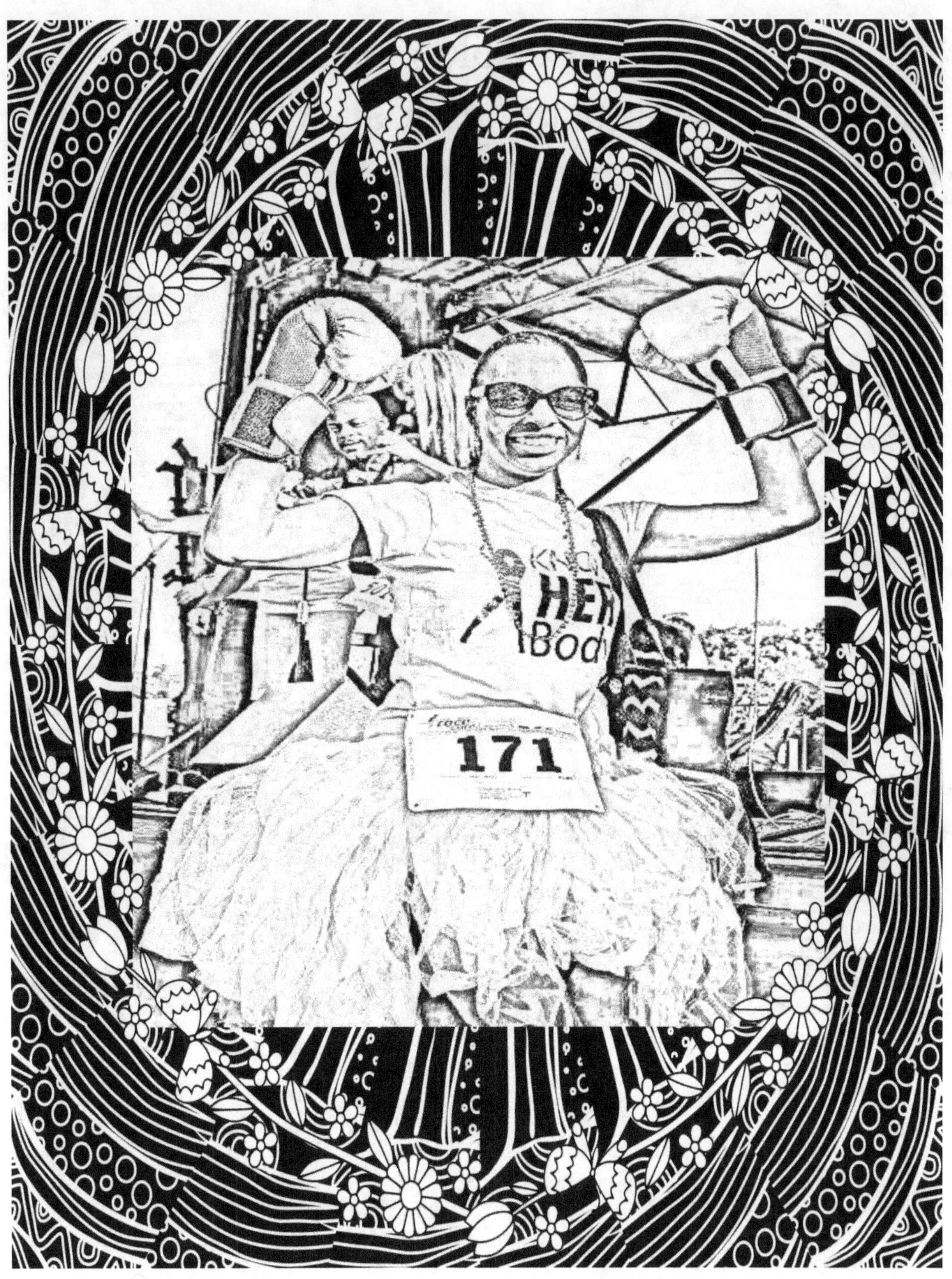
171

For more coloring books, journals, and planners for breast cancer survivors visit:

FightLikeaGrownAssWoman.com

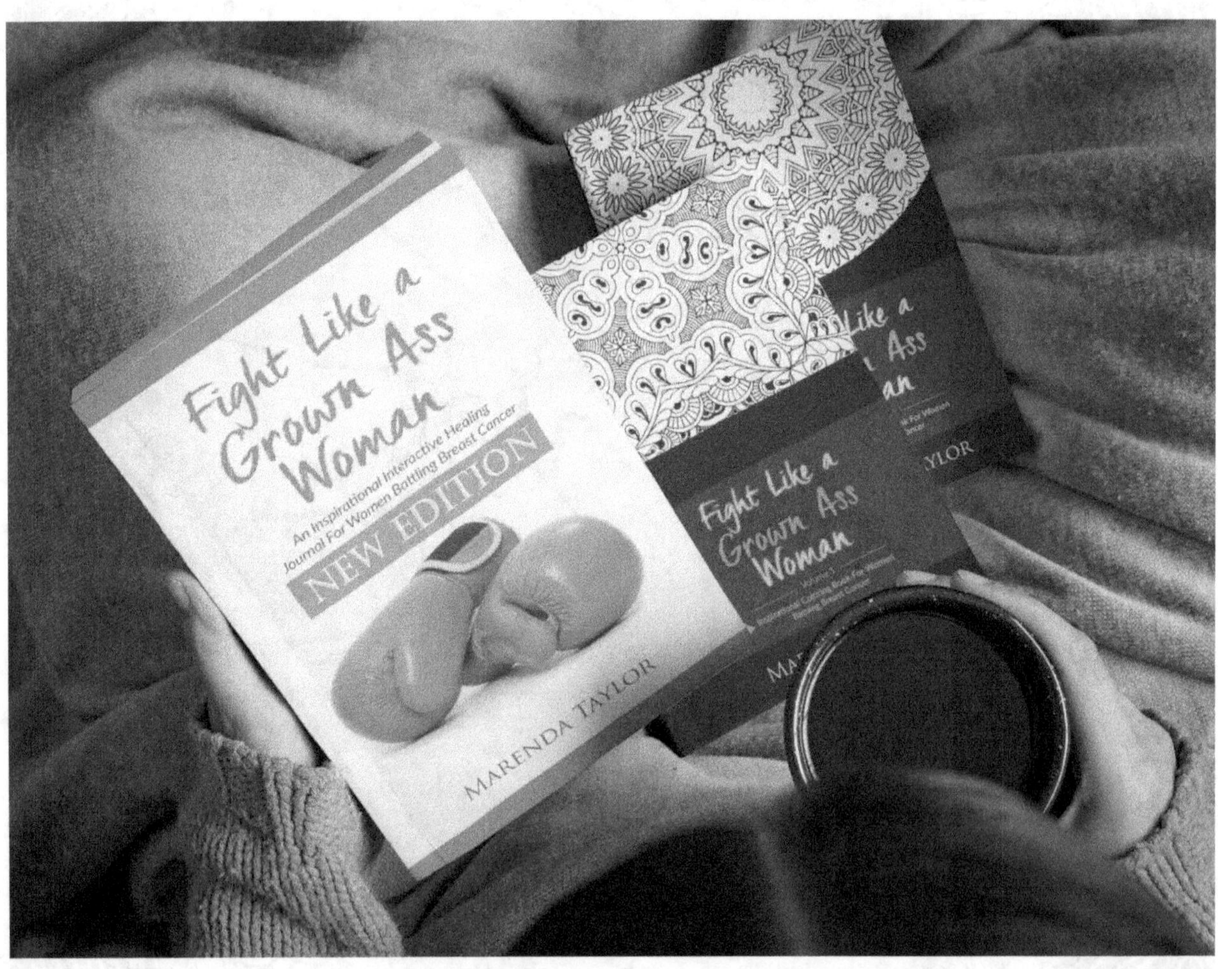

Get Stylish Survivor Wear here:
InspirationQueen.com

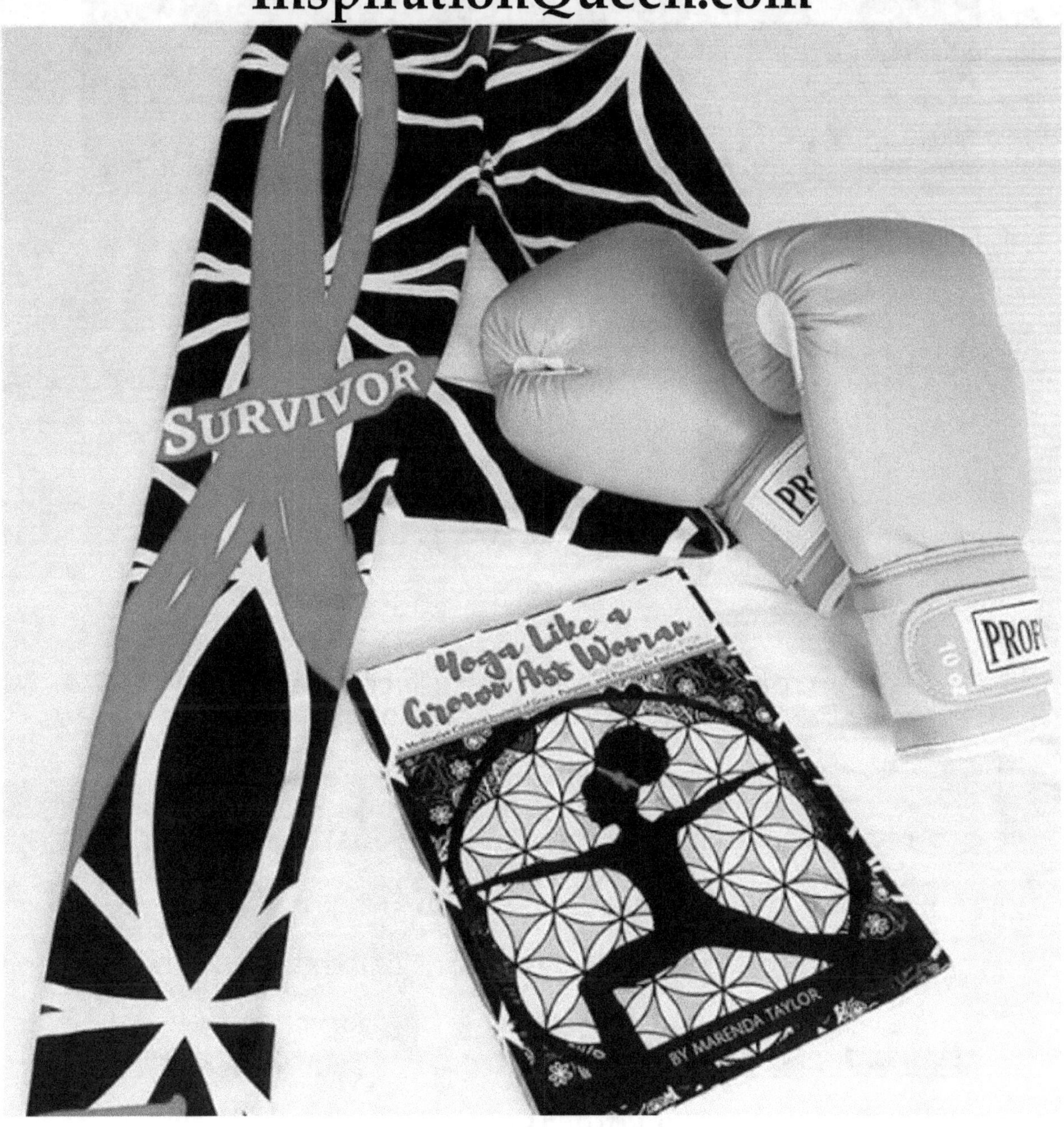

Be sure to add all of these great UpwardAction® Media titles to your business building library.

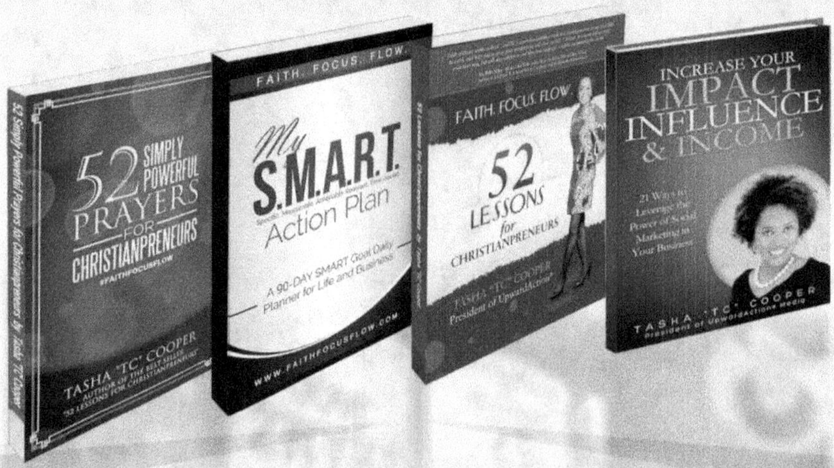

Increase Your Impact, Influence & Income with Social Marketing

52 Lessons for Christianpreneurs

My SMART Action Plan: A SMART Goal Planner for Business and Life
(Available in 30 and 90 Day Editions)

52 Simply Powerful Prayers for Christianpreneurs

All titles by Tasha "TC" Cooper

These and other great professional development resources are available at
www.UpwardActionMedia.com

FightLikeaGrownAssWoman.com